HANDMADE MEDICINES

Simple Recipes for Herbal Health

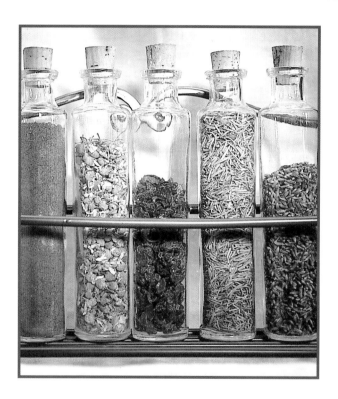

CHRISTOPHER HOBBS, L.AC.

In this book, the author is not prescribing herbs or other substances for any medical condition, but rather describing their historical and current use. The material in this book is not a substitute for individual advice from your health-care practitioner. The author and editors of this book emphasize that a total program for health, which can often effectively include an herbal regimen, is th only lasting and sure way to assist the body in its healing processes.

Handmade Medicines: Simple Recipes for Herbal Health
by Christopher Hobbs

*Photo props courtesy of Fox Ryde Gardens, Loveland, CO, and
    The Cupboard, Fort Collins, CO.*
Cover design: Dean Howes
Photography: Joe Coca
Text copyright, 1998, Christopher Hobbs
Photography copyright, 1998, Joe Coca and Interweave Press, Inc.

Botanica Press is an imprint of Interweave Press

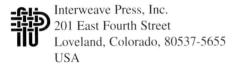 Interweave Press, Inc.
201 East Fourth Street
Loveland, Colorado, 80537-5655
USA

Printed in the United States of America

First Printing: 7.5M:298:VGN

DEDICATION

To Beth for everything, and for helping me keep at least one foot on the ground and on my path, and to Rosemary, for helping to keep my heart open to the plants and so many incredible people.

ACKNOWLEDGMENTS

I would like to gratefully acknowledge all the herbalists and wise women, past and present, whose dedication and love of healing herbs have made this book possible.

Because no herbalist is an island, I am fortunate to have learned skillful ways of preparing and using herbal remedies from so many fine herbalists over the years, especially Herbal Ed Smith and Brian Weissbuch, L.Ac. Through the insights of many herbal friends I have deepened my appreciation for the spiritual and healing ways of herbs on other levels, particularly Rosemary Gladstar; Michael Tierra, L.Ac.; Gabriel Howearth; James Green; and Cascade Anderson.

Herbs are the benevolent medicines and allies of all creatures: two-legged, four-legged, and winged. May we not forget their sacrifice or take their gifts lightly. May we remember to protect their homes, families, and tribes with all our best intentions.

INTRODUCTION

WHY MAKE YOUR OWN HERBAL MEDICINES? Won't that be dangerous? Won't you need lots of high-priced equipment? And what about skill? You'll need to know a lot to make your own medicines—right?

Actually, making safe and effective herbal medicines is well within your reach, for the tradition of making medicines at home with healing plants is both ancient and worldwide. In many cultures everyday ailments have been treated with handmade herbal medications for generations; in fact, only recently have medicines *not* been made in the home.

Are herbal medicines safe? Yes, when prepared and used as recommended by an experienced herbalist. I've used the simple recipes and procedures in this book for years in my clinic of herbal medicine; they have helped others to better health by working with the body's healing process, not against it. The equipment is simple and probably in your kitchen now; a food dehydrator is the most complicated piece of machinery mentioned here, and it's not necessary, just convenient.

Gentle and slow-acting, most herbal medicines do their work without jarring the body's systems or requiring constant monitoring, as many pharmaceutical drugs do. Modern medicine relies primarily upon chemical, synthetic molecules to formulate the drugs we are routinely offered. In contrast, handmade medicines offer safe, gentle complexes of healthful ingredients from nature that stimulate the body's own healing capabilities, encouraging health from within.

When you make your own medicines, the ingredients are of your own choosing. The medicine may be specific for a single problem—a nagging cough, for instance—or you can make a medicine that contains several ingredients. You needn't worry about adulterations such as pesticides, filler ingredients, or additives. The medicine contains only what you choose.

If growing and enjoying beautiful plants is part of your life, you'll find yourself appreciating them in a new, exciting way. As you learn about their healing properties, you'll see your garden as not only lovely, but a source of positive healing support as well.

With this book, you can make unique herbal products to benefit yourself and your family. By planning your own herbal medicine chest and filling it with fragrant and useful extracts, oils, creams, and salves, you can keep the healing power of herbs at your fingertips.

When I became interested in herbal medicines about thirty years ago, *The Modern Herbal*, written by Maude Grieve in 1931, guided my first acquisition of herbs: valerian, chamomile, rosemary, cayenne, and ginger. Of course Mrs. Grieve's book was outdated, but at that time no one was teaching about herbs or offering courses by mail, and local college officials wouldn't have imagined having a class about herbs. The topic was so obscure that my friends and neighbors, soon considered me weird and gave me the Havabanana award as the most radical health fooder and natural medicine user in the community.

In 1984, I was considering ways of making a living with herbs. At about the same time, I learned about milk thistle and wanted to try it for my liver, which had been weakened by hepatitis many years before. Finding none available commercially, I harvested the seeds from local wild milk thistle and made my own extract. After taking this preparation for several months, I noticed a positive difference in my digestive health.

To share this helpful information with others, I began a small herb company, which grew to a national firm in only five years. In 1989, my partner Beth and I decided to sell the company because its business aspect took us away from what we loved best: being with the plants and writing and teaching about them.

Over the years, I've made numerous herbal extracts and preparations and taught many others the art and science of herbal medicine-making. I continue to enjoy harvesting herbs and making preparations for our own use and to give to my patients. From this clinical, personal, and always hands-on experience, I have developed the medicine-making techniques and herbal formulas in this book.

Whether your interest in herbs comes from a deep appreciation for nature's power to heal, from a grandparent or ancestor who used herbs, a chance encounter with someone's bottle of echinacea tincture for your sore throat, a desire to be self-sufficient with your medicine and healing process, skepticism about high-tech pharmaceuticals, or simply the promise of less expensive but safer health care, this book is for you.

TABLE OF CONTENTS

8
Chapter 1: Ancient Herbal Medicine-Making

13
Chapter 2: Why Herbal Medicines Work

18
Chapter 3: Finding Healing Herbs

50
Chapter 4: Preparing Herbs for Use

64
Chapter 5: The Recipes

113
Table 1: Useful Solvents for Herbal Medicines

117
Resource Directory

119
Index

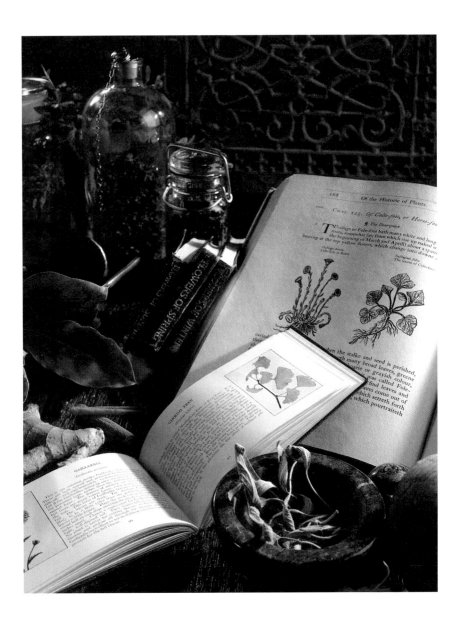

CHAPTER 1

ANCIENT HERBAL MEDICINE-MAKING

SAFEGUARDING HEALTH AND HEALING have always been human concerns, and for at least 5,000 years people have devised potions, elixirs, salves, and other herbal preparations against illness and misery. The Sumerians, residents of a southern Babylonian kingdom of city-states in what is now Iraq, left written records of medicinal herbal preparations that are strikingly similar to those we use today.

The Egyptian culture developed at about same time as the Sumerian culture. Their healers built a sophisticated body of knowledge about herbs and their uses. In this, the Egyptians surpassed the Greeks, who embraced the practice of using diet, healthy living habits, and other natural methods to treat disease and preserve health.

We know of the Egyptians' skill in making medicinal preparations from medical scrolls discovered in tombs during the nineteenth century. The most magnificent, the Ebers Papyrus, is a medical teaching text nearly sixty feet long. It was written during the Eighteenth Dynasty, or about 1550 B.C.

Translated around the turn of the twentieth century, the Ebers Papyrus contains 829 prescriptions for internal diseases and injuries such as broken bones. Specific dosage information is given for 599 maladies. Scientists who study these texts have identified dozens of herbs mentioned in the scroll. Egyptian physicians ministered to their patients' ills with herbal preparations that are similar to those available today. They made salves and ointments from oil and beeswax and prescribed them for burns, bites, and wounds. Patients were told to mix their herbal powders with beer and wine, because physicians understood the power of alcohol to carry the active ingredients of herbs into the bloodstream. Honey was used to make bitter and acrid herbs taste better, and it was mixed with flour to form pills. An Egyptian tomb painting from the fifteenth century B.C. shows the preparation of herbal ointments: workers blend, stir, and cook the ingredients into an ointment.

The herbal recipes recorded in the Ebers Papyrus came from even earlier times; ancient medical writers often refer to *old* writings from which they have borrowed. Some of the Ebers Papyrus prescriptions are said to date from the time of Usaphais, a king of the First Dynasty (prior to 3,000 B.C.). Another recipe was allegedly prepared for Shesh, mother of King Teti, during the Sixth Dynasty (ca. 2,500 B.C.).

The power of the ancient medicine-makers echoes to the present day. Remedies that originated with the Egyptians and Assyrians were used through the heydays of the Greeks and Romans, adapted amidst the Persian flowering of medical and pharmaceutical advances of about 700 to 1400 A.D., and studied in the early Italian medical schools at Padua and Salerno beginning in the fifteenth century. Many European formularies, from the eighteenth century to present times, arrange herbal recipes according to symptom or illness, as did their Egyptian forebears of 2,500 years ago.

By the 1930s, however, Western medicine was turning toward synthetic drugs as replacements for herbal preparations, although the use of herbs continued in some areas. In the United States, the 1936 edition of the *National Formulary*, a record of drugs prescribed and allowed for sale in pharmacies, included numerous herbal extracts such as echinacea, saw palmetto, dandelion, blue cohosh, and Oregon grape root. Most herbs were dropped in later editions, and by 1995 only a few remained.

Fortunately, the art of medicine-making remained alive and well in many other countries of the world, especially Germany and most Asian cultures, and these continuous traditions are valuable resources for herbalists today. The 1997 edition of the *U.S. Pharmacopoeia* will include, for the first time since the 1930s, an expanded list of herbs that reflects the medical profession's response to the public's growing interest in the benefits of herbal medicine.

You can join this fine human tradition by reading and using this book. You, like ancient healers, hold in your hands a record of remedies that reaches back through the ages. You have available, as they had, plants that heal. Your harvest of wild or cultivated herbs can fulfill the basic human desires to ease pain, preserve health and vitality, and promote long life. And, like those who have gone before, you can gather this healing power, prepare it, and use it for the comfort and improved health of yourself and those around you.

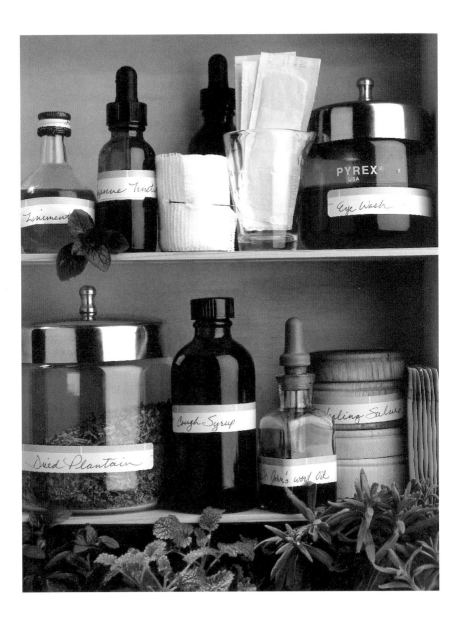

CHAPTER 2

WHY HERBAL MEDICINES WORK

KNOWING ALL THE INNER WORKINGS of plants is not essential for making effective and safe herbal medicines, but knowing something about the nature of plants will help you make and use high-quality preparations.

By weight, plants are composed primarily of starches and sugars (soluble fiber) that store energy, and cellulose and lignin (insoluble fiber) that give plants shape. Like our own bodies, plants also contain a large proportion of water. Together, these elements—the primary constituents—make up more than 95 percent of a plant.

The secondary constituents comprise the remaining 5 percent of the plant, and among these are medicinal ingredients. Despite sometimes occurring in very tiny amounts, medicinal constituents can have powerful actions. For instance, the traditional digestive herb gentian contains a compound so bitter that a single drop of the extract can be tasted in a gallon of water.

Constituents occur in different proportions in different parts of the plant. For instance, flowers are typically high in sugars like sucrose, and all above-ground plant parts contain coloring pigments like anthocyanidins and flavonoids, the plant's own "sunscreens" that protect its genetic material from ultraviolet-light damage. Seeds contain unique fats to provide energy for the fast-growing sprout, and roots act as storehouses for food and medicines. Because the useful properties of plants are unevenly distributed, it is important to learn where the medicinal constituents are concentrated in each plant you may wish to use. Another important consideration is the timing of harvest, for the potency of constituents varies during the plant's life cycle.

The objective of preparing herbs for medicinal use is to separate the active constituents from the rest of the herb, concentrate them, and efficiently carry them throughout the body. Not all constituents dissolve willingly into a single solution, however; alcohol is an excellent solution for some constituents, but others are better dissolved in plain water. Thus it's helpful to learn which solutions suit which herb.

THE SAFETY AND USE OF HERBS

What about the safety of the herbs themselves? Science has revealed little about most plant constituents although some, such as caffeine, have been thoroughly studied. When scientific studies are done, however, the effectiveness of herbal preparations is typically consistent with the herb's history of use *when the herb is prepared and taken properly.* When herbal treatments are compared to treatments with pharmaceutical drugs, fewer and milder side effects usually are recorded for the herbal compounds. In addition, herbal preparations are often less expensive than pharmaceuticals. Although scientific study has not yielded volumes of information on medicinal herbs, it has confirmed a good deal of the herbal tradition and pointed out some excellent reasons for using herbs for healing.

Like all medications, herbs can be harmful when misused or taken carelessly. One's individual physical condition and current medications can bear upon which herbs to take and which to avoid. For instance, echinacea stimulates the immune system, so it should not be taken by those who have immune-system disorders such as multiple sclerosis, lupus, or rheumatoid arthritis; stimulating a misdirected immune system could lead to a worsening of the patient's condition. Finally, any individual can develop an idiosyncratic allergic reaction to an herb, just as to tomatoes or eggs.

How can one feel confident about taking handmade medications? If the following situations are present, you should consult a qualified herbalist or carefully investigate particular herbs before taking them:

- Pregnancy, anticipated pregnancy, or nursing
- A course of medications or other drugs taken
- Presence of chronic illness
- History of allergies
- Extreme youth or advanced age.

PLANNING YOUR HERBAL MEDICINE CHEST

In choosing the herbs to keep at home, consider the contents of your medicine cabinet. Most people keep on hand pain relievers, cold medicines, digestive remedies, something to promote sleep, and products for wounds, rashes, or burns. Prescription drugs are probably in there, too.

Herbs can treat most everyday medical and health needs, including injuries. Following are some of the most common conditions and injuries for which you may seek a drug or healing preparation. I have listed some common over-the-counter products for each condition along with healthy herbal alternatives.

Pain Relievers

Common headaches	Aspirin, ibuprofen	Valerian tincture, white willow bark
Migraine	Prescription drugs	Feverfew
Muscle aches	Ben-Gay	Cayenne liniment, wintergreen oil
Canker sores	Campho-Phenique	Calendula tincture

Cold Medicines

Colds	Aspirin, Dristan	Echinacea, ginger tea, garlic
Coughs	Vicks lozenges, Robitussin syrup	Wild cherry bark, mullein
Congestion	Robitussin syrup	Eucalyptus steam, sage
Sore throat	Sucrets lozenges	Thyme, echinacea
Fever	Tylenol or aspirin	White willow bark
Cold sores	Campho-Phenique	Lemon balm cream

Digestive Remedies

Heartburn	Tums, Rolaids	Licorice

Nausea	Dramamine	Ginger, peppermint
Intestinal cramps	Alka-Seltzer	Chamomile, peppermint
Ulcer	Prescription drugs	Licorice, St. John's wort infused oil

Skin Problems

Bleeding	—	Yarrow leaf and tincture
Dry skin, chapped lips	Chap-Stick	Creams, salves of calendula, plantain
Pimples	Noxzema	Burdock root, dandelion root
Infections	Neosporin Cream	Echinacea tincture, goldenseal
Rash	Campho-Phenique	Calendula salve

Injuries

Bruises, sprains	Sports creams such as Aspercreme	Salves, creams, oils of calendula, arnica
Minor burns	Campho-Phenique, A & D Ointment	Salves, creams of calendula, plantain
Cuts	Bactine Ointment	Powdered cayenne or yarrow, burdock

Stress Symptoms

Insomnia	Sleep-Eze	Valerian, California poppy
Tension, anxiety	Aspirin Prescription drugs	Kava kava St. John's wort

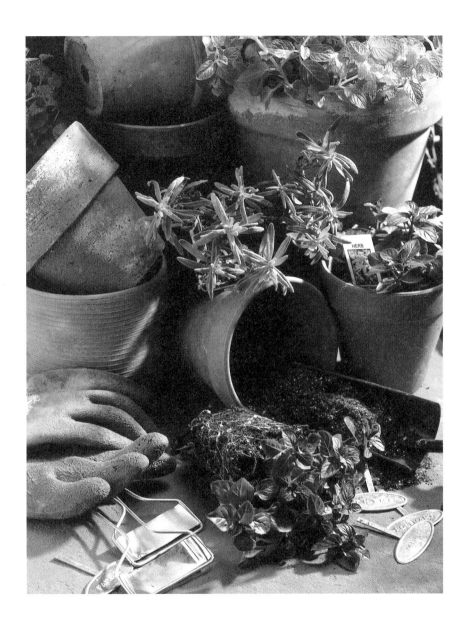

CHAPTER 3

FINDING
HEALING HERBS

MAKING HANDMADE HERBAL MEDICINES requires a reliable source of high-quality herbs. The freshest, best herbs may be those you grow yourself in your garden. You also may be able to wildcraft fresh herbs, harvesting them carefully to preserve their medicinal qualities. The most reliable source of some useful herbs, however, may be the local herb shop or a mail-order herb supplier.

I encourage you to grow or harvest at least one herb and use it to make your own healing preparations. Your appreciation and awareness of the beauty and healing essence of herbs growing in their natural homes are powerful connections to the bounty that nature provides.

GROWING A MEDICINAL HERB GARDEN

Not so long ago, the only medicine available came from herb gardens or wild land. By the Middle Ages and the Renaissance, the increasing size of cities made herbal medicine gardens quite practical, and a tradition was born. Sometimes communities cooperated to grow a medicinal garden; all worked in the garden, and all benefited from the herbs it produced. This is an idea whose time may have come *again;* several families in an ordinary Los Angeles neighborhood recently organized a community food and medicine garden, sharing both labor and harvest and improving relationships in the neighborhood.

An herb garden need not be large, but it should suit your personal needs for healing. Do you lead a hectic life with too much stress? Consider a calming garden filled with chamomile, lemon balm, wild lettuce, and California poppy. From such a garden could come delicious fresh teas, tinctures to settle the nerves and bring on sleep, and dried calmatives to last the winter. If cold weather seems to be one long ordeal of colds, sniffles, flu, and congestion, try a garden of echinacea, garlic, lemon balm, thyme, yarrow, and peppermint; they will provide antiviral action, boost the immune system, fight congestion, and reduce fever.

Many medicinal herbs grow happily in pots, making the traditional garden unnecessary. Container gardening, an old art that has become popular again, is particularly suitable when one has no access to a sunny gardening patch. A few pots can yield useful medicinal herbs for a variety of ailments.

When purchasing plants and seeds for your garden, be sure that you bring home the medicinal variety of the particular herb; closely related plants may differ significantly in their medicinal properties. Plant names can be confusing, too; a good example is the pot marigold. Its scientific name is *Calendula officinalis,* and it is a very different plant from the common marigold, *Tagetes,* whose ruffled yellow and orange blooms light up gardens from spring until frost. For this reason, the scientific names of the choice medicinal varieties are given here. If you have trouble finding the correct varieties or species, plants and seeds for medicinal herbs can be purchased by mail from growers listed in the Resource Directory.

THE TOP MEDICINAL GARDEN HERBS

The amazing abundance and usefulness of medicinal herbs make allocating garden space a real challenge. The following herbs have been chosen because each has a proven track record of safety and effectiveness when used medicinally, the seeds or small plants are easily found, and the plants are not overly picky about their environment. Each appreciates well-drained soil that has been loosened with organic material. All grow best in a sunny place, but some will tolerate shade. Two applications of a well-balanced garden fertilizer will assist the plants to maximum growth. Make the first application in early spring when new growth appears, and the second when buds begin to form.

Burdock *(Arctium lappa)*. This plant is a biennial; that is, it requires two years to reach maturity. Harvest the seeds of the mature plant in summer and dig the root in late summer.
Medicinal Uses. A poultice of fresh or dried leaves is antibiotic and helps heal abscesses and boils. The seeds may be used to brew a tea that is cleansing and diuretic. Fresh burdock root is a strengthening nutritive tonic when sliced into soups and stir-fries; the Japanese use it often and call it *gobo*. Tea and tincture of the

dried root cool and calm the liver while stimulating the flow of bile and other digestive enzymes.

Calendula *(Calendula officinalis)*. Harvest "pot marigold" flowers just before they burst into bloom and remove any that are spent to encourage even more prolific production.

Medicinal Uses. Calendula flowers, dried or fresh, may be used to make a tea that reduces digestive difficulties. The tea can also be used as a vaginal douche against yeast infection. Tinctures or oil infused with the flowers helps heal burns, rashes, and other injuries.

California poppy *(Eschscholzia californica)*. A Western United States native, this herb willingly adapts to many other conditions. Sow California poppy seed early in the spring and harvest the entire plant at bloom. The plant grows easily and reseeds well.

Medicinal Uses. California poppy is a safe, effective sedative that relieves mild pain and anxiety without the chemicals that make the opium poppy dangerous; in fact, it's safe for children. Used primarily as a tincture, California poppy helps relaxation and brings on refreshing sleep. The root is the most potent part.

! *Seek expert advice before taking California poppy if you are taking antidepressants, pregnant, or anticipating pregnancy.*

Cayenne *(Capsicum frutescens)*. Once established, cayenne pepper plants revel in heat and tolerate drought. Harvest the ripe red peppers with the stems on. To dry them in a traditional way, thread a large, sharp needle with string or fishing line. Pierce the pepper stems with the needle, string them up, and dry in well-ventilated shade.

Medicinal Uses. Always remove the seeds from the peppers when using them medicinally. Taken internally, cayenne protects the heart and blood vessels by invigorating and warming the circulation. It improves digestion and acts as a decongestant. Applied externally in an infused oil, it makes a good liniment for aching muscles.

! *Reduce dose or discontinue cayenne if it causes gastrointestinal discomfort. Wear rubber gloves when handling the peppers or powder; never rub your eyes or touch other delicate skin areas before washing your hands.*

Chamomile *(Chamomilla recutita).* Chamomile isn't a fussy plant. Early summer blooming signals the beginning of harvest; removing the tiny flowers just prior to bloom stimulates more blossoms.

Medicinal Uses. The tea of both Roman and German chamomile is antispasmodic and calming; it soothes bowel cramps and eases nausea and indigestion. Oil infused with chamomile and applied directly to the skin reduces inflammation. In tincture, chamomile flowers are useful against irritable bowel syndrome. Chamomile is safe for both adults and children.

! *Pregnant women may use German chamomile, but not Roman chamomile.*

Comfrey *(Symphytum officinale).* Comfrey grows vigorously, even aggressively, in most garden soils. It starts from seed in spring or from root division in autumn. Harvest the leaves and flowering tops in summer.

Medicinal Uses. Compresses of comfrey leaves and flowering tops encourage the healing of sprains and broken bones as well as burns and rashes. The poultice is helpful for the same conditions. I recommend using only the leaves as a tea for only a week or two at a time. Ulcers and irritable bowel conditions often respond to this regimen.

! *Pregnant or breastfeeding women should not use comfrey internally, and everyone should avoid internal use of the roots.*

Dandelion *(Taraxacum officinale).* Dandelions, as everyone knows, start easily from seed sown wild or by hand, and once the long, tough tap root is established, the plant is practically permanent. All parts of the plant are useful.

Medicinal Uses. In the early spring, harvest the fresh green leaves and enjoy them in salads for their tonic and diuretic properties. (Unlike many other diuretics, which flush potassium from the body, dandelion leaves replace potassium.) The leaves also act as a bitter digestive, stimulating juices in the stomach that help break down food. Later in the spring, pluck the yellow blooms just as they open and make dandelion wine. Finally, during the early autumn, dig and dry the root. Prepared as a tea, dandelion root cleanses the liver and helps resolve skin problems. For extra cleansing power, combine dandelion root with burdock root.

Echinacea *(Echinacea angustifolia, E. purpurea).* Wildcrafted nearly to extinction in some areas, this hardy, drought-tolerant, native perennial thrives in the garden. Given a boost of fertilizer now and then, it's spectacular. Harvest the blooms as they open, the leaves as needed, and the root the third or fourth year.

Medicinal Uses. Water- or alcohol-based preparations of the flowers, leaves, and roots stimulate the immune system and reduce symptoms of colds, flu, and infection. Tea of the flowers, leaves, or roots is beneficial, but the root is most powerful in *E. angustifolia*.

Preparations of echinacea are most beneficial when taken intermittently. For instance, when early cold symptoms appear, take echinacea for a week or ten days, then set it aside for a few days. If symptoms persist, resume taking echinacea another week to ten days, then discontinue it.

Fennel *(Foeniculum vulgare).* Tall, sweet-smelling fennel grows easily in temperate zones but requires attentive watering. It is best started from small plants. Seeds are harvested in the fall. The feathery leaves can be used as a culinary herb, and Mediterranean cuisine often features the bulb as a vegetable.

Medicinal Uses. Fennel seeds help the digestive system by easing gas pains and cramping. A gargled infusion of the seeds will help a sore throat. Fennel tea increases breast-milk production.

Feverfew *(Tanacetum parthenium).* Naturalized throughout temperate zones, feverfew starts easily from cuttings or seed and requires little care. Harvest fresh leaves as needed, and harvest the whole plant when it is in full flower.

Medicinal Uses. To prevent migraine, eat two or three fresh leaves daily, disguising the taste with other foods. Whole-plant preparations include tinctures and capsules. For some, feverfew eases the pain of arthritis.

! *Avoid feverfew if pregnant or anticipating pregnancy.*

Garlic *(Allium sativum).* Grown nearly worldwide, garlic is easy to cultivate. The clove, planted in the early spring, produces a bulb that is pulled up late in the summer.

Medicinal Uses. Before the discovery of modern antibiotics, garlic was often used to treat infections and wounds, both internal and external. The infused oil or fresh clove can be applied to skin injuries for its antibiotic and antiviral effects. An earache can be relieved with a few drops of warm garlic oil in the ear. Taken internally, garlic supports the heart and blood vessels and lowers serum cholesterol and blood pressure. It acts against lung and bronchial infections.

! *The raw clove pulp can cause redness and irritation if left too long on sensitive skin. If garlic causes digestive upset, discontinue.*

Goldenseal *(Hydrastis canadensis).* A Native American remedy, goldenseal is becoming rare in the wild in some states. Propagated by root division or seed, it requires a moist habitat with deep mulch and shade. Three-year roots are dug in the autumn and dried.

Medicinal Uses. A celebrated tonic and anti-inflammatory, goldenseal is antibacterial, astringent, and bitter. An infusion of the powder is effective against yeast infections or heavy menstrual flow when used as a vaginal douche. The tincture, taken orally, regulates mucus flow throughout the body and relieves digestive inflammation. Filtered and used as an eyewash, it reduces eye irritability and redness.

! *Goldenseal can be toxic when overused. Avoid altogether during pregnancy and nursing or if high blood pressure is present.*

Hops *(Humulus lupulus).* Cultivated throughout Europe and increasingly in the United States for flavoring beer, hops grows easily. The scaly flowering clusters, or strobiles, are gathered in the autumn and used fresh or dried.

Medicinal Uses. Hops is useful in relieving nervous tension and anxiety, especially for people with heart palpitations from overwork or stress. It encourages refreshing sleep and calms and improves digestion. Most often taken in a tea, it can also be tinctured (the most potent extract will come from a tincture of fresh strobiles). A sachet of the strobiles and other calming herbs such as lavender releases a soothing aroma that encourages relaxation. The tea also promotes milk production in breastfeeding mothers.

Horehound *(Marrubium vulgare).* Start this hardy perennial from stem cuttings or small plants. Gather the leaves in the spring, and during the rest of the warm season, prevent it from overtaking the rest of the garden.

Medicinal Uses. By stimulating mucus production, this herb relieves dry coughs and wheezing. It is most often prepared as a tea, syrup or candy. It is also an expectorant and cough suppressant.

Lavender *(Lavandula officinalis)*. Adaptable in temperate zones, lavender requires a sunny spot for best growth. While the plant blooms during its first year, it reaches its full size in the second or third year. The flower heads are collected in midmorning just at bloom and dried; several harvests are possible over the summer growing season. Several varieties of lavender are available; I have always favored the classic scent of English lavender, but Spanish and French lavender are also wonderful.

Medicinal Uses. Most people agree that the scent of lavender is soothing, and it has long been used to lighten the spirits. A tea of the flowering tops, added to the bath, relaxes the muscles and improves the mood. The undiluted essential oil is excellent for burns. To treat indigestion or nausea, add lavender to after-dinner tea and take along with ginger. A sleep pillow that includes lavender along with hops and other calming herbs contributes to restful sleep.

Lemon balm *(Melissa officinalis)*. Capable of growing three to four feet tall if given adequate space and sun, lemon balm is a hardy perennial. Once established, the plant is care-free. Tender leaves can be regularly harvested as the plant fills out and becomes a delightful addition to any garden. The above-ground parts are harvested for medicinal purposes.

Medicinal Uses. Lemon balm has long been cultivated for its calming properties, but recent research has focused on its antiviral uses. Tea or cream prepared with the herb aids healing when applied directly to cold sores or other herpes lesions such as shingles.

The juice of fresh lemon balm leaves, rubbed on the skin, soothes insect stings or bites. Very companionable with chamomile in tea, lemon balm eases indigestion as well as irritability and nervousness. Tinctures, infused oils, and juices of the plant are similarly useful.

Marshmallow *(Althaea officinalis)*. Best started from small plants, marshmallow likes moisture; once established, however, it tolerates some drought. Harvest the above-ground parts at bloom; dig the roots in autumn.

Medicinal Uses. An infusion of the root, taken at the first suggestion of urinary tract infection, often prevents the problem from developing. This preparation also aids digestive ills such as irritable bowel syndrome or colitis, in part because it is gently laxative. Its mucous membrane-soothing properties also make it useful in treating bronchial irritation, stomach ulcers, and asthma. A flower infusion, applied directly, soothes damaged skin. A decoction of the root, prepared in a cream, helps heal boils.

! *Marshmallow, taken internally, may delay the absorption of pharmaceuticals; check with your health-care provider.*

Mullein *(Verbascum thapsus)*. Mullein is a biennial that sets a rosette of leaves the first year, flowers the second year, and then usually dies. In milder climates, it can last another year. Spikes that can become 6' tall carry the flowers, and these, as well as the furry leaves, are harvested in the summer.

Medicinal Uses. Mullein leaves make a good-tasting tea for strengthening the lungs and loosening mucus. It is the best, safest, all-around respiratory tonic, and can be used continuously for any health problems involving the respiratory tract, including bronchial asthma. The flowers, infused in oil, make an excellent preparation for relieving ear infections. When applied to the skin, mullein flower oil aids wound healing.

Peppermint *(Mentha piperita).* For the gardener, the challenge of peppermint is not growing it—that's easy—but containing its growth. Easily established in most soils, this mint tolerates shade and drought and spreads aggressively by both underground and aboveground runners, so cut it back severely in spring, fall, and as needed during the summer. The leaves of peppermint can be harvested as needed during the summer for medicinal use in teas, oils, and tinctures as well as pleasant nibbling and culinary uses.

Medicinal Uses. Peppermint-leaf tea settles the stomach and helps reduce gas and bloating. It relieves intestinal cramps, especially when combined with other herbs such as chamomile that also aid digestion. Peppermint oil, taken in enteric-coated capsules, soothes the smooth-muscle spasms of irritable bowel syndrome. For nausea, peppermint and ginger are combined in tea.

As an inhalant, peppermint breaks up congestion to make breathing easier. During colds and flu, it soothes inflamed throats and eases coughs. Its antiseptic qualities help heal minor skin wounds.

Plantain *(Plantago major; P. laceolata).* This tough perennial is usually harvested from the wild, but giving it a place in the garden assures that its first-aid help will be available when needed. It is widely naturalized in temperate zones; sown in the garden, it requires little attention and readily self-seeds. The leaves are harvested as needed.

Medicinal Uses. Plantain leaves, applied fresh or as a dried-leaf poultice to a wound, speed healing and reduce inflammation of cuts, burns, bites, stings, and other external injuries. Internally, a tea is useful for lung problems, infection, and bowel and urinary tract irritation or inflammation. While the plantain leaves have a strong antibiotic effect, other parts of the plants do not.

Rosemary *(Rosmarinus officinalis).* Originally a Mediterranean plant, rosemary likes sun, well-drained soil, and protection from harsh winds or extreme cold. It is hardy and drought tolerant, but doesn't mind sitting in water. Harvest the tender new sprigs as needed.

Medicinal Uses. Rosemary is an excellent tonic that can be used regularly to invigorate circulation and the nervous system. For those recovering from chronic illness or surgery, it lifts the spirits and encourages healing. A tea or tincture of the plant, taken internally, can help start the menstrual flow. The tea, added to the bath, aids sore muscles and arthritic pain while stimulating circulation.

! *Do not use rosemary preparations if you are pregnant or anticipating pregnancy.*

Sage *(Salvia officinalis)*. Sage can be started from seed, but it is best grown from small plants or rooted cuttings. Drought-tolerant once established, it requires little care, but often lives only three or four years. Harvest the leaves in summer.

Medicinal Uses. Antiseptic and astringent, fresh sage or a poultice of dried leaves helps heal wounds. Use the tea for a digestive and nerve tonic, or, with the addition of a little honey, for coughs and colds. Gargle the infusion for a sore throat. Sage tea also reduces hot flashes and helps dry mothers' milk. And the tincture can be sprayed under the arms as a natural deodorant that also reduces sweating.

! *Do not take therapeutic doses of sage when pregnant. Culinary levels of the herb are safe.*

St. John's wort *(Hypericum perforatum)*. Seeding or root division result in hardy perennial plants that typically bloom about St. John's Day, June 24. Harvest the top 12" of the plant as the flowers open.

Medicinal Uses. St. John's wort is well recognized as effective against mild to moderate depression when taken as a tincture or powdered extract. Less well known are its effectiveness against ulcers when the infused oil is taken internally and its antiviral effects; its anti-inflammatory properties make the infused oil effective in treating external wounds, bruises, and irritations as well. The oil, massaged into a sore area, aids in healing damaged nerves.

! *If you are taking antidepressants, do not take St. John's wort preparations internally without expert advice. Avoid overexposure to sunlight when taking the herb; it can cause increased sensitivity to sunburn.*

Stinging nettle *(Urtica dioica)*. Yes, it stings, and raises a rash, too. Use protective gloves when harvesting; collect tender tops in the spring as tonic vegetables. During flowering, take the leaves and flowering tops. Dig the rhizomes and roots in the fall. The green parts of the plant lose their sting when steamed like any other green, leafy vegetable.

Medicinal Uses. An excellent cleansing herb, stinging nettle is a diuretic and astringent. The root decoction is taken for enlarged prostate, and the tincture helps allergies, skin conditions, and arthritis. Some use the nutritious leaves in soups. Two or three cups a day of infusion of the leaves act as a tonic and blood builder.

Red raspberry *(Rubus idaeus)*. This thorny canefruit is usually grown in temperate climates for its fruit, but the leaves, harvested in the early summer, are useful as well. Raspberries tolerate shade but require moisture for best production.

Medicinal Uses. A tea of the leaves can be used as an eyewash in cases of mild infection and for a mouthwash when sores are present. The tea also eases and speeds labor when taken regularly throughout pregnancy. When diarrhea is a problem, a decoction of the leaves is helpful.

! *Discard any dried or drying leaves that seem moldy or discolored, and dry the leaves thoroughly before storage.*

Thyme *(Thymus vulgaris).* I grow at least ten varieties of thyme for both culinary and healing purposes and especially like caraway, lemon, and English thymes. It prefers light soil, but adapts well to heavier soils that are enhanced with compost or other loosening materials. Gather the small, tender sprigs as needed throughout the spring and summer.

Medicinal Uses. Thyme can be taken as a tea, tincture, or an oil. Because thyme is antiseptic, it can be applied to the skin to relieve infection. The herb makes a tea effective against sore throats and upper respiratory tract infections. It is also used in cough syrups and candies.

! *Use caution with thyme essential oil; it is very irritating to the skin. Only a few drops are needed in syrups or baths.*

Yellow dock *(Rumex crispus).* Perennial yellow dock can grow up to 5' tall. Tender leaves are harvested in the spring, and the yellow root is dug in the fall. Harvest some of the wild seeds to plant in your garden.

Medicinal Uses. The young tender greens make a good vegetable when steamed. The tea or tincture of the yellow roots can help build the blood, cleanse the liver, and remove heat and dampness in the colon. Long used as a gentle laxative, the herb helps heal bowel irritations, vaginal yeast infections, and urinary tract infections.

! *Individuals with a history of kidney stones should use caution with this herb.*

Yarrow *(Achillea millefolium).* Of all the lovely varieties of yarrow, the plain white-blooming *millefolium* is the most reliable for medicinal purposes. This easygoing, creeping perennial's roots spread underground. The above-ground parts are harvested when the plant is in flower.

Medicinal Uses. A powder made of the dried leaves is an ideal styptic to stop the bleeding of shaving cuts or other minor wounds; a poultice of the fresh or dried leaves, pressed to a wound, stops bleeding and reduces the chances of infection. A pinch of yarrow powder sniffed up the nose often stops nosebleed.

Yarrow possesses antiviral, cleansing, and sweating properties that are useful against colds and flu. In addition, it improves circulation, and particularly benefits varicose veins. Both tea and tincture, taken internally, promote the menstrual flow and reduce the pain of uterine cramps.

! *Do not take yarrow preparations if pregnant or anticipating pregnancy.*

WILDCRAFTING

If you don't have the time or space to grow your own herbs, you may be able to harvest some from vacant lots or wild areas. In fact, some herbs are so common that once you recognize them, you see that they're all around you. Be aware, however, that successful wildcrafting requires knowledge of the herbs, information about harvesting regulations, and adequate preparation.

First, nearly every government entity regulates the use of the lands it controls, including the picking of wild plants. Investigate and respect the regulations that govern any public area that you wish to explore for herbs. Picking plants is forbidden in some areas, while other areas are open to harvesting, with or without a permit.

If you wish to harvest herbs from private property, avoid trouble by contacting the landowner before searching for herbs. Trespassing can result in arrest.

Contact your state department of agriculture or division of wildlife to learn which plants are endangered or protected. Some popular herbs, such as goldenseal, black cohosh, and ginseng, are becoming rare in some states. In parts of the world where medicinal herbs are routinely used, some are extinct in the wild. Learn to distinguish native herbs that are rare or scarce. Our natural heritage deserves respect and preservation.

Select harvesting sites that are at least 100 yards away from roads, depending on the quantity of traffic. Avoid also agricultural areas where pesticides and herbicides might be used and industrial areas with factories and mills. Particulate air pollution can enter the plant through the leaves, and some plants absorb toxins such as heavy metals from the soil.

Hone your skills in identifying and observing plants. Correctly identifying wild herbs is essential, for many have poisonous or less active look-alikes. Others are endangered, and some are protected species that cannot be picked under any circumstances. Further, if you harvest the wrong part of the plant, or harvest at the wrong time in the plant's life cycle, your effort may be wasted along with the plant.

Close observation improves skills in selecting wild plants for harvest. For instance, Ryan Drum, a conscientious wildcrafter with over twenty years' experience, takes great care in observing and harvesting wild plants.

He once told me that red clover heads are in their prime for only a day or two. The flowers mature from the bottom up on the head. As the tiny individual flowers open, they are at their peak. The maturing unopened flowers are also useful. But once the flowers have been pollinated, their medicinal quality declines within an hour or two. A prime flower head has only a few flowers dried and hanging down at the bottom; most of the other flowers are nearly mature or blooming. Drum's close knowledge of medicinal plants allows him to harvest excellent plants while maintaining the plant population.

When you have selected an area in which to search for herbs, begin planning your harvesting by deciding how much herb you need. Once in the field, it is easy to become excited by the process and harvest more herb than you can use, leading to waste. Pack proper tools, such as shovels, spades, and clippers, and use cloth bags, paper bags, or buckets to carry the herbs. Plastic bags accumulate moisture and heat, accelerating the breakdown of the herb material.

When you find the medicinal herb you seek, select only one in ten for harvest if you are taking up roots. If you are clipping flowers or fruits, take only one flower or fruit of three, or clip the flowering heads from one of three plants. If there are only a few plants, leave them be.

Harvest each plant with thankfulness for its gift of life and health, for thoughtlessly grabbing a plant does not lead to powerful medicine. We could learn much from Native Americans, many of whom harvest medicinal plants with reverent ritual and prayer. They avoid harvesting the oldest plants—the grandfathers and grandmothers—and the youngest plants. Healthy, middle-aged plants that are free from insect damage and discolored leaves are harvested, and the plant population survives to provide another harvest in the future.

Each region of the United States has its own wealth of medicinal herbs that are native to the area or naturalized. To investigate the location and use of these plants, consult your local library or bookstore, or speak with an herbalist or botanist knowledgeable about the region's plants. I recommend *A Field Guide to Medicinal Plants: Eastern and Central North America* by Stephen Foster and James Duke, as an outstanding resource. For the Western United States, Michael Moore's *Medicinal Plants of the Pacific West* and *Medicinal Plants of the Desert and Canyon West* are excellent. The following herbs can be found frequently in temperate areas.

Burdock *(Arctium lappa).* This plant, recommended above for the garden, is often found growing wild. Use the wild plant the same as a cultivated one.

Chicory *(Cichorium intybus).* The roasted root of chicory has long been used as a coffee substitute, and it is a mild, bitter digestive tonic. Harvest the root in the autumn.

Dandelion *(Taraxacum officinale).* Use wild plants as you would cultivated ones, but avoid dandelions that have been sprayed with herbicides.

Hawthorn *(Crataegus oxyacantha, C. monogyna).* This shrub or small tree has proven to be effective in treating cardiovascular ailments. Tincture of the flowering tops or berries is used to lower blood pressure and increase blood flow to the heart. Flowering tops can also be used to treat and help prevent circulatory disorders. The berries, which contain digestive enzymes and fruit acids, make a tea that strengthens the digestion. The herb is the most widely respected heart tonic in Western herbalism.

Horsemint *(Monarda punctata)*. The aboveground parts of this plant, gathered when in flower, make a tea effective in relieving nausea and other digestive difficulties. Applied externally as a poultice, the herb relieves the pain of arthritis or other inflammations.

! *Avoid if pregnant or anticipating pregnancy.*

Milk thistle *(Silybum marianum)*. Milk thistle grows in sunny, open places and reseeds easily. Collect the seeds in autumn and prepare them in a tincture to protect or heal the liver.

Mullein *(Verbascum thapsus)*. Recommended also for the garden (above), this plant is found in many temperate areas.

Plantain *(Plantago major, P. lanceolata)*. Widely naturalized in the United States, this plant is also recommended for the garden (above).

Red clover *(Trifolium praetense)*. Widely cultivated as fodder and seen in waste areas, this herb's flowers contain estrogenic ingredients that may be useful in treating menstrual difficulties. Harvest the blooms at the beginning of full flower. As a blood purifier, red clover tea is helpful for cleansing programs and skin conditions.

! *Avoid if pregnant or anticipating pregnancy.*

Self-heal *(Prunella vulgaris)*. The tea of the leaves and flowers can be gargled to relieve sore throat or fevers from flu. In ointment, it helps heal skin wounds, hemorrhoids, and varicose veins.

St. John's wort *(Hypericum perforatum)*. Widely naturalized throughout the United States, this plant is also recommended for the garden (above).

Stinging nettle *(Urtica spp.)*. This herb is a common native plant throughout temperate zones and is also recommended for the garden (above). Different species grow in every region. Use protective gloves when gathering.

Willow *(Salix spp.)*. The bark of this tree contains a chemical forerunner of aspirin. A tincture or decoction of white willow bark helps relieve fevers and pain. Harvest the tender bark only from newly fallen or pruned twigs and branches. Harvest the bark in the early spring before flowering.

Wild garlic *(Allium spp.)*. The many species of wild garlic can be used like cultivated types recommended for the garden.

Wild lettuce *(Lactuca virosa)*. The dried juice of this common plant's above-ground parts makes an excellent sedative or sleep aid.

Wild onion *(Allium* spp.). Use wild species just as the cultivated one.

Yarrow *(Achillea millefolium)*. Watch the summer roadsides for white wild yarrow; it has the same healing properties as its cultivated cousin.

So many additional healing herbs can be found in every climate that it would be impossible to list them all. To discover the herbs that grow wild in your area, consult your librarian, botanist, or local herbalist.

Buying Herbs

Most herbalists, even dedicated gardeners and wildcrafters, purchase medicinal herbs from time to time because particular plants can't be obtained any other way. Ginger and kava kava, for instance, grow only in tropical climates, so buying them from reliable sources is the only option for most. Establishing a garden or wildcrafting takes time and must be done in season; perhaps the best reason to purchase herbs, however, is a quick start to making handmade medicines.

Fortunately, many natural products shops and herb stores carry a variety of medicinal herbs, as do a growing number of natural-foods cooperatives and other alternative purchasing groups. Herbs are usually available in several forms, such as fresh, dried, powdered, and so on. To bypass the time and preparation of gardening or wildcrafting, draw up a list of the medicinal herbs you want to use and investigate the resources in your community.

Everyone has access to herbs by mail order. If your search of community resources does not yield all the herbs you'd like, phone an herb company with credit card in hand. Soon your herbs will arrive at your door. In the Resource Directory are listed several excellent herb suppliers. I am familiar with these companies and trust them to provide high-quality herbs.

When you purchase herbs, feel free to ask lots of questions before you make your decision. Some sources offer certified organically grown herbs, but others make no such guarantee. Ask about testing of the herb material (which usually verifies that the herb is, in fact, what the company represents it to be), the methods by which it is prepared, and how old the herb material might be.

When bulk herbs arrive, check them by smelling them and examining them closely. Dried flowers such as calendula should be close to their original color—orange, in this case. Green plants like peppermint should be vibrant green, not brown, and the smell of many herbs should be fresh and aromatic—very much like the fresh herb. If any herbs you have ordered smell musty, or look brown, dirty, or lifeless, feel free to return them.

You may also find that retail herb outlets and mail-order sources offer equipment, tools, and supplies that you will find useful for preparing your handmade medicines. A collection of catalogs from such companies can be a handy resource as you continue making medicines. Purchasing the following herbs is the most practical way of getting them, because they grow in very specific climates.

Arnica *(Arnica montana)*. Arnica, a native of the European and North American mountains, is becoming scarce in the wild. Prepared as an infused oil or as tincture used in lotions and ointments, arnica is helpful in healing bruises, sprains, and strains.

! *Arnica is poisonous if taken internally, and can cause irritation if used on broken skin.*

Astragalus *(Astragalus membranaceus)*. An Asian plant, astragalus strengthens the immune system, improves digestion and energy, and helps overcome anemia. The prepared root slices look like tongue depressors and are widely available in herb shops or from Chinese herb dealers. Astragalus can be used over a long period and is an excellent addition to homemade soups or stews.

! *Do not use during acute infections.*

Cinnamon *(Cinnamomum verum)*. The world's tropical highlands are the home of this warming herb. The inner bark of the tree can be purchased in "sticks" or ground. For medicinal use, purchase the sticks and grind them in a coffee grinder as needed. Cinnamon stimulates the digestion and is beneficial for those recovering from illness. A hot cinnamon tea is warming and a mild decongestant. Tincture of the bark is antibiotic and antifungal.

! *Avoid medicinal doses of cinnamon if pregnant or anticipating pregnancy; amounts typically used in cooking, however, are harmless.*

Elder *(Sambucus nigra)*. Both the flowering tops and berries of the elder tree have medicinal properties. For cold symptoms such as cough, congestion, and fever, the tea or tincture of flowering tops promotes sweating and cleansing and is antiviral. The berries are mildly laxative, and a decoction eases the pain of rheumatism.

Fenugreek *(Trigonella foenum-graecum)*. The seeds of this herb stimulate uterine contractions. Fenugreek is nourishing, stimulates the appetite, and acts as a cleanser on the liver and bowels. It is also useful during convalescence and against anorexia. The seeds may stabilize blood sugar levels.

Flax *(Linum usitatissimum)*. The tiny seeds of flax can be used whole, in which case they are an effective, cleansing bulk laxative. Ground, they are rich in fatty acids; as a poultice, flax seeds relieve chest congestion and inflammation and help heal boils.

! *Flax seeds, often called linseed, are used in the preparation of oils used in furniture finishing and oil painting. Never use such oils either internally or externally; they may be toxic. If you are gathering flax seed, be aware that immature seeds may also be toxic.*

Ginger (*Zingiber officinale*). This tropical plant is cultivated for its root, now widely available in supermarkets as well as natural products stores. It is sold fresh, powdered, and crystallized. Ginger relieves postsurgical nausea as well as motion and morning sickness. It calms the intestines and reduces gas and cramping and serves also as a mild laxative. By stimulating circulation, ginger warms the extremities.

! *Ginger tea made from fresh roots is safe during pregnancy; dried roots are not.*

Ginseng (*Panax ginseng*). Taken as a tonic, especially for the elderly, ginseng is essential in Traditional Chinese Medicine. Although the plant grows in temperate zones, over harvesting has made it difficult to find; cultivating it, however, is successful. Preparations should be taken for short periods of about six weeks when stress relief, digestive support, or extra energy is needed. Ginseng strengthens the immune system to prevent chronic infection.

! *Do not use excessive amounts of red Korean or red Chinese ginseng if you have a chronic infection or inflammation like arthritis. It can be overheating and stimulating. People under 40 should use American ginseng or Siberian ginseng, which promote energy but are not excessively heating.*

Kava kava *(Piper methysticum).* A tropical plant that plays a ceremonial as well as practical role in Pacific Island cultures, kava kava root relieves anxiety and mild pain while relaxing the muscles and promoting refreshing sleep. The tea can help heal urinary infections, and it combines well with other relaxing herbs such as valerian and St. John's wort.

Licorice *(Glycyrrhiza glabra).* This herb, native to Asia and southeastern Europe, soothes the stomach lining and relieves inflammation elsewhere in the body. Thus it is useful against ulcers, colitis, and inflamed joints. The tea or diluted tincture is also a gentle laxative. It is part of many adrenal support formulas.

! *Anise, not licorice, provides the flavor of licorice candy; it has no medicinal value. If suffering from high blood pressure, use licorice only on the advice of a trained herbalist.*

Psyllium *(Plantago* spp.). Rich in mucilage, psyllium seed is used extensively as a laxative and can help irritable bowel syndrome, Crohn's disease, colitis, and hemorrhoids. Soak half a teaspoon of seeds in water for fifteen minutes to an hour; take the whole dose at bedtime, along with more water. Many benefit from first taking small doses of psyllium and working up to a full dose.

Turmeric *(Curcuma longa).* Tropical turmeric is usually available as powdered root or extract in tablets. It is a powerful anti-inflammatory and protects the liver. A weak tea can be taken against stomach upset, and a poultice of the powder, applied to skin eruptions such as eczema, soothes discomfort. The tincture can be taken daily.

! *Do not use turmeric medicinally if pregnant or anticipating pregnancy.*

Valerian (*Valeriana officinalis*). Valerian is extremely effective in relieving the symptoms of stress and nervous anxiety: insomnia, tight muscles, panic, headache, and heart palpitations. Menstrual cramps and irritable bowel syndrome may also respond to treatment with it. Preparations of the dried root have a strong, unpleasant odor; those from the fresh root have a more sweet, spicy smell and are better relaxants.

DRYING AND STORING FRESH HERBS

Whether you grow, purchase, or wildcraft your fresh herbs, any that are not used right away should be dried. When the plants are harvested, an enzymatic reaction begins that eventually destroys their medicinal constituents. Drying, boiling, or exposure to alcohol stops the reaction.

If working with fresh herbs, examine them carefully and remove any plant parts that are damaged or discolored. Clean them carefully with a cold-water rinse and pat them dry. Because heat and sunlight are the enemies of medicinal constituents, dry your herbs in an airy place where sunlight cannot strike them. A kitchen or laundry area where they will be subject to moisture, or a closed garage that heats up, won't produce the best result. Instead, choose a screened porch, an open garage, or even a shed that has good airflow and stays cool to warm. Use a small fan to circulate the air if necessary. Leafy herbs, their stems tied into small bundles, can be hung upside down and shade dried. If you are drying several types of herbs simultaneously, label the bundles.

Shade-drying is also effective for heavier plant material. To dry roots or bark, chop the material into thin, angled slices. Whole flowers such as calendula and chamomile can be dried, too. Place these thicker plant materials in a single layer on a cookie sheet lined with paper towels or, better yet, a drying screen made of window screen stretched over a wooden frame.

Check your drying herbs every day or so, because over-dried plants are weak in medicinal constituents. Plants are dry when small stems snap easily when bent and leaves crunch between your fingers. Plants that are too dry lose their color and are very brittle.

A food dehydrator is handy for drying small quantities of herbs, especially leaves separated from their stems. A fast and efficient food dehydrator can become the home herbalist's favorite tool.

STORING HERBS

Dried herbs are best stored in airtight, lidded jars that are kept in a pantry or cupboard where little light penetrates. Whole dried herbs keep best, followed by sliced or coarsely cut herbs. Powdered herbs have the shortest shelf life. It's best to store the whole dried herb and cut, grind, or powder it when you are ready to use it.

Label the jars clearly, especially if you combine herbs. Add the date of storage; dried herbs are best used within six months, and two years is the maximum storage time.

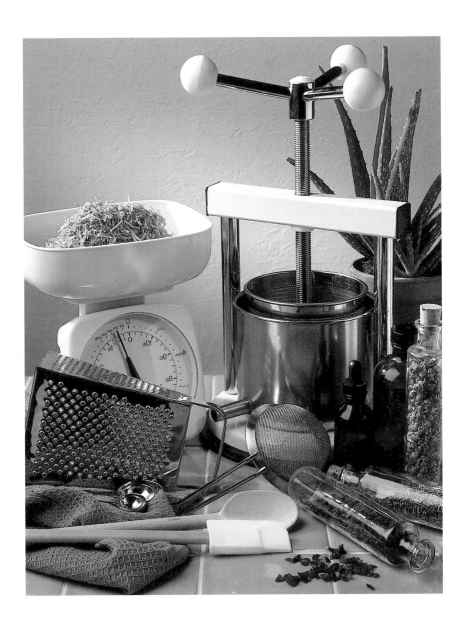

CHAPTER 4

PREPARING HERBS FOR USE

Now that you've grown, wildcrafted, or purchased your healing herbs, what's the next step before they become medicine?

In some cases, none—the herb comes from the plant or the store ready to eat. Fresh young dandelion leaves are easy to add to a salad for a digestive tonic; crystallized ginger can be nibbled out of the bag or box to soothe nausea.

Using other medicinal herbs can be as easy as boiling water, for many herbs are effective either fresh or shade-dried and steeped in warm or hot water. Such teas—also known as infusions or decoctions, depending on their strength—can be drunk, used in an herbal bath, or applied to the skin in a compress. Herbs can also be infused into oils and vinegars for skin and muscle remedies and culinary uses.

Still other herbs require a bit more preparation to isolate and concentrate their medicinal components. To make the recipes in Chapter 5, you'll use solvents— glycerin or alcohol, (with or without water)—to attract and hold the healing substances from these plants. Once the extraction process is complete, the spent

REMEDIES FROM THE SPICE RACK

It's surprisingly easy to use tasty, healthful herbs to support your ongoing good health. Just be sure they're reasonably fresh.

Cayenne *(Capsicum annuum)* invigorates and warms the circulation, improves digestion, and acts as a lung decongestant. Sprinkle cayenne powder into soups, stir-fries, and tomato-based sauces.

Cinnamon *(Cinnamomum zeylandicum)* remedies nausea and indigestion and works against diarrhea, too. Sprinkle the powder on applesauce, yogurt, toast, oatmeal—it's tasty with many foods.

Garlic *(Allium sativum)* is helpful against colds, infections, and intestinal parasites. It also keeps the blood thin and lowers blood pressure. This valuable herb can be used fresh, powdered, granulated, or as an oil.

Ginger *(Zingiber officinalis)* supports digestion, relieves nausea, and stimulates circulation. Painful digestion, colic, and diarrhea respond to ginger, taken fresh or in tea.

Turmeric *(Curcuma longa)* improves digestive function overall and is effective against diarrhea and inflammation. Some studies indicate that turmeric protects against cancer. This useful herb is a prime ingredient in curries and other Indian dishes; its warm yellow color brightens meals.

plant is ready for the compost bin and the extract can be used as it is or it can become an ingredient in another herbal medicine. These extracts are known as tinctures when the solvent is alcohol or alcohol and water, and glycerites when the solvent is glycerin.

EQUIPMENT

The making of medicinal extracts requires only a few pieces of equipment, and most are probably in your kitchen now.

Blender or Grinder

Using a blender or grinder reduces the dry or fresh plant material to the smallest possible particle size and increases the surface area that is exposed to the solvent, resulting in a more complete extraction with less waste. Some herbs, such as ginseng, are expensive—up to $600 per pound—so getting the best possible extract is important.

While any good blender will be useful, it's best to use one with a very strong high-speed motor. A Vitamix has an extra-strong motor, and it is reversible to help untangle herb roots and stems from the blade. The reverse option also leads to a more complete breakdown of the plant material. Blenders are made in different sizes; if you're replacing yours, you may wish to purchase a large one. A Waring blender with a one-gallon capacity is a good choice.

A small seed or coffee grinder such as a Moulinex grinder is handy for finely powdering small quantities of dry seeds, root slices, and leaves. It often yields a finer particle size than a blender.

Food processors can be useful for shredding fresh roots, seeds, and leafy material. They are best, however, for chopping herbs prior to placing them in the blender or grinder. For larger jobs, like shredding burdock roots or dislodging the seeds from milk-thistle heads, you might want to consider a small garden-compost shredder.

Pots 'n Pans

There's always some debate about the type of pots and pans best used when working with herbs. I recommend that you use only uncoated stainless steel or glass cookware. Examine the bowls and utensils you wish to use; if they're cracked, discard them. Avoid aluminum pans that can interact with herbs, giving discolored or off-tasting products.

Pyrex glass is my favorite material in which to cook herbs and herb oils. Coffee pots that are made of good quality heat-resistant glass are excellent because the glass does not interact with the herbs. It's also easy to gauge the progress of the extraction process by observing the color of the developing extract. I judge the strength of a decoction, for instance, by its dark rich color. Double boilers are also useful for melting wax and warming ingredients without overheating or scorching them.

Some people like crock pots for making infused herbal oils. The gentle, steady warmth of the pot increases the medicinal concentration of the final oil. A crock pot suitable for this purpose should allow the temperature to be turned to about 100 degrees Fahrenheit (37°C.).

Weights and Measures

Some of the ingredients used in making herbal remedies—such as beeswax—are typically measured and sold by the pound or ounce, so a small kitchen scale may come in handy. If you bring a few pre-weighed items with you on your shopping trip, you'll be able to check the scales' accuracy, whether you look for one at an upscale kitchen store or your favorite second-hand emporium.

Containers and Labels

For working with medicinal herbs, canning jars are invaluable. They are relatively inexpensive, widely available, and come in many sizes. I use quart or half-gallon jars for storing and extracting herbs. When dried herbs or extract solutions are placed in the clean jars and the lids twisted down tight, all external elements are sealed out.

For bottling smaller quantities of herbal liquids, purchase amber Boston rounds—the small, brown-glass jars with droppers that are commonly used to package commercial herbal liquids. They come in sizes holding from one ounce to eight ounces of liquid, and they're very handy.

You'll want to label the contents of your herb jars, including the ingredients and the date you created them. Include instructions for taking the herb and any warnings that apply. Adhesive labels can be found at any discount or office supply store; some also carry decorative label sheets that can be used in your computer's printer.

Food Dehydrator

A food dehydrator is a good investment for the home herbalist. It will dry flowers, leaves, root slices, and other herb parts quickly while preserving valuable constituents and color. Culinary herbs like oregano, basil, and thyme can be quickly dried, too. Herb juices and cooked-down herb extracts can be dried and powdered using the nylon fruit-leather tray inserts that come with the dryer or as an accessory.

If you plan to make powdered extracts, purchase a dehydrator with an adjustable fan speed and temperature.

The Main Squeeze

Although a juicer is not essential to making herbal extracts, it increases the types of herbal products you can make. These machines extract the juice from fresh herbs, which can then be taken fresh, or dried and used later. A hand-operated herb press helps squeeze the liquid from tinctures and infused oils. Especially when working with expensive herbs, getting those last few drops from the mixture is worthwhile. To obtain one, check with your local natural-products store or Resource Directory listings.

MEDICINE-MAKING TECHNIQUES

Some medicinal herbs transfer their benefits to distilled water better than to oil or alcohol. On the other hand, the healing ingredients in a number of herbs dissolve into several solvents. Herbalists can spend years learning the best solvent for each herb by studying old pharmacopoeias, the *United States National Formulary*, and old pharmacy texts. See Table 1 on page 113 for a list of frequently used herbs and their solvents; this information is based on my thirty years of study, making herbal preparations, and clinical practice.

Teas, Infusions, and Decoctions

When water is the solvent, purified, distilled water is best. Tap water and other types of bottled water may contain unwanted chemicals such as chlorine, as well as minerals and salts that are unnecessary and potentially damaging to the herbs' medicinal qualities.

Warm-water infusions preserve the maximum amount of volatile components such as essential oils. They also protect the integrity of fragile plant substances like the polysaccharides in echinacea leaves. Combine one part plant material with four to ten parts of room-temperature water, depending on the density or absorbent properties of the herb. Grind the mixture in the blender until smooth and let it steep for eight to twelve hours. Strain the mixture and discard the herb. Drink the infusion in one-cup doses, three to six times daily.

Sun tea is also a gentle infusion. Place cold water and herbs in the proportions above in a clean, clear glass jar with a lid. Put the closed jar in a sunny place and leave it until the tea is strong enough to suit your tastes, up to four or six hours. Strain the herb from the tea and enjoy the drink at room temperature or cold.

Hot-water infusions are often used in making medicinal teas from leaves or flowering tops. Typically, use one pint of boiling water for every ounce of dried herb. Pour the boiling water over the herb and let stand, covered, for fifteen to twenty minutes. Strain the herb from the liquid and discard the herb. Take the tea in one-cup doses at least three times daily, up to six cups. For very light and fluffy herbs, like mullein or chamomile blossoms, increase the amount of water.

Decoctions are made from the hard or woody parts of the herb, such as bark or root. The constituents of roots, barks, twigs, and chips are best extracted in water by simmering in an uncovered pot for forty-five minutes to one hour; use about one ounce of herb to ten ounces of water. After simmering, strain the liquid and discard the herb.

The resulting liquid can be drunk at once or refrigerated for later use. I often make up to two quarts of a decoction at once; if I drink a cup both morning and evening, it lasts four days. Don't keep herbal teas longer than this, as they can ferment.

In making a decoction, about 25 percent of the liquid will be lost through evaporation and herbal absorption. If you want to make a quart of tea, start with five cups of water to four ounces of herbs.

Double Decoction. If you're working with costly herbs such as ginseng or astragalus, it's cost-effective to double-decoct the herbs. After the first simmering, described above, strain the herbs and set the tea aside. Add more fresh water to the herbs, but only about one-quarter of the amount used during the first simmering. Simmer again for about thirty minutes, let cool fifteen minutes, and strain, squeezing out as much liquid as you can from the herbs. Blend the two teas together, and the batch is ready to use. In my experience, a third simmering is not productive; the first two get 90 percent or more of the medicinal constituents from the herb.

Light Decoction. For lighter barks, such as willow or cinnamon bark, and some hard leaves like horsetail or horehound, make a light decoction by simmering the herbs, covered, on the lowest heat possible for ten to fifteen minutes. Leaving the lid on the pot prevents the escape of volatile constituents like essential oils. Let the mixture steep for another ten or fifteen minutes, then strain and use or refrigerate as above.

Preserving Infusions and Decoctions

In these busy times, it's often convenient to make a large batch of medicinal tea, using only part of it at once and saving the rest for later— but not beyond the four-day limit for keeping tea in the refrigerator. One of the easiest ways of preserving medicinal teas is freezing, which extends its usefulness up to three months. When the tea is cooled, pour it into ice-cube trays and freeze; then pop the cubes out and store them in heavy plastic freezer bags, using as needed.

Our favorite herbal ice cubes are echinacea cubes, which are very effective against sore, inflamed throats due to cold or flu. A favorite summer flavor is lemon; ice cubes of lemon balm, lemon verbena, or lemon thyme make nearly any herbal ice tea taste more refreshing. We've also made raspberry-leaf tea ice cubes for pregnant women; this herb strengthens uterine contractions. The new mothers report that the crushed cubes were welcome during labor.

Medicinal teas can also be dried for even longer shelf-life and greater convenience. You can make your own dried teas at home with little effort and almost no equipment. Besides being potent, safe, and alcohol-free, dried teas are relatively cheap to make. If stored

About Essential Oils

Infused oils and essential oils are not the same and must not be used in the same ways. Essential oil is obtained from the herb itself by distillation, and a great amount of herb yields only a small amount of oil, accounting for the high price of true essential oils. Essential oils are extremely concentrated and should never be taken internally without professional advice; many are toxic. For external use, they must be well diluted with other oils in order to avoid skin irritation.

Infused oils, on the other hand, are much gentler and safer. Made by soaking herbs in vegetable oil, they carry the medicinal properties of the herb without harshness. Infused oils may be enhanced by small additions of essential oil, but they are in no way comparable to essential oils.

in a cool place out of direct sunlight, they have a shelf life of up to a year or more, and they can be powdered and placed into capsules.

Infused Oils

Herbal infused oils are vegetable oils that contain active ingredients from herbs. These oils can be used to help soothe rashes, sunburns, and other skin irritations. Some are useful against the pain of strains, sprains, and sore muscles, and they speed the healing of such injuries.

Herbal infused oils are made by blending dried (or sometimes fresh) herbs into the oil, using as much herbal material as possible. The mixture steeps, or macerates, for two to three weeks. It should be stirred or shaken daily. After careful filtering, the finished oil can be bottled and refrigerated. You can also use a crock pot to make your oils more rapidly. No matter how they're made, infused oils can be used directly or mixed with beeswax to make healing herbal salves. Chapter 5 contains recipes for oils, creams, and salves.

Tinctures, Glycerites, and Vinegars

Some herbs will give up their medicinal constituents only to alcohol, liquid glycerin, or vinegar. Of these three solvents, alcohol is by far the most efficient, but not everyone is able to take herbs in this form. In these cases, glycerites and vinegars, taken at higher doses than tinctures, are indicated.

Tinctures

For prompt results in treating acute conditions and adjusting or stimulating the energy of the body, I often recommend alcohol-based tinctures. Alcohol extracts medicinal constituents efficiently and carries them into the bloodstream quickly.

For home use, tinctures can be made with 100-proof vodka or pure grain alcohol. One hears of herbs being tinctured in other alcoholic beverages such as rum and brandy; these concoctions are often promoted as tasting better than regular tinctures. These beverages, however, contain pigments, flavoring compounds, sugars, and other components that diminish their effectiveness in drawing out the medicinal components of herbs, so the medicines made from them may be weaker than those made from 100-proof vodka, and some may be much less effective.

Pure grain alcohol, distilled from corn, is superior to vodka as a solvent. Distilled water is sometimes added to grain alcohol to adjust the drawing power of the solution for various purposes. For instance, the medicinal constituents of milk thistle are soluble only in alcohol, so a solution that is very high in alcohol is best. The phytosterols in ginseng, however, are more water soluble, so a mix of water and alcohol is appropriate.

Tinctures are made by grinding up dry or fresh herbs in a solution of alcohol and water; the liquid is called the *menstruum*. Commercial tinctures are often made with one part herb to five parts menstruum, which is notated (1:5); that is, one cup of herb requires five cups of menstruum.

Glycerites

When glycerin is used to extract herbal constituents, the resulting product is called a glycerite. Herbal glycerites are a good choice for people who don't want alcohol; some parents choose these solutions for their children because the preparations can be stirred into juice.

Glycerin is also kind to the skin. It moisturizes without creating an oily feel or leaving a heavy residue, making it a popular ingredient in skin-care products. Another property of glycerin is its ability to bring together oils and tinctures in a smooth, easily applied blend, so it is a good medium for combining various forms of medicinal herbs to suit oneself. For example, one might combine glycerin with tincture and infused oil for healing and an essential oil for scent to create a unique product. Glycerin is a weaker solvent than alcohol; it can dry the throat if taken straight.

Vinegars

Vinegar, a weak solvent, is not often used as the only solvent to make a liquid extract, but it is sometimes added to alcohol, glycerin, or water to draw out certain constituents and help preserve the final product.

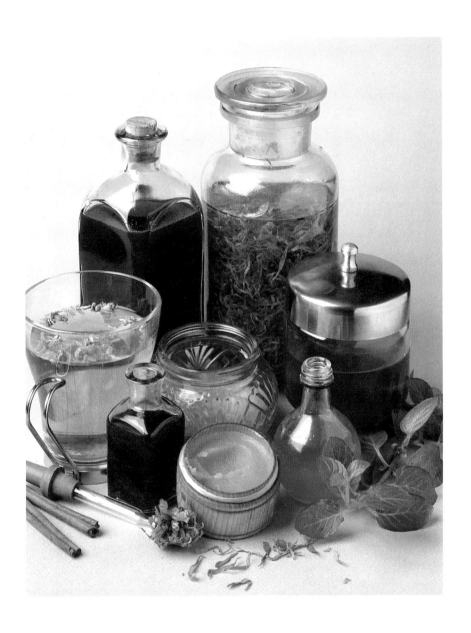

CHAPTER 5

THE RECIPES: COMBINING HERBS FOR HEALING

Although this chapter is about ways to combine, preserve, and use herbs, it's easy to forget how simple herbal medicine can be. If it's spring, summer or fall—or you live in a warm climate—there are probably healing plants growing not too far from where you're reading this book.

When it comes to making herbal medicines, especially teas, most people use dried herbs. The majority of extracts of herbs such as saw palmetto and ginkgo, now rapidly becoming popular, are also made with dried herbs. One might assume, then, that dried herbs are superior to fresh; in fact, many people have asked me whether they could use fresh herbs because the only herbs they had ever seen were dried.

Actually, fresh herbs are the most potent and desirable form of healing plants. My friend "Herbal" Ed Smith says, "You wouldn't eat brown lettuce, so why take brown herbs?" He refers to the color of many commercial dried herbs, even ones that started out as green, red, yellow, and other fresh colors.

When an herb is dried, it loses varying amounts of its active constituents, depending on how it was dried and how long it was stored before use. Fresh herbs, however, contain all the medicinal activity that nature intended, with minimal enzymatic breakdown. Fresh herbs usually require only a quick rinse under cold water and a check for insects prior to use. Be sure to discard any plant material that is discolored or damaged.

While fresh plants often have the maximum amount of biochemical activity, herbalists commonly feel they also have something extra that is hard to measure—"essence," or "Qi." When an herb is fresh and consumed directly from the earth, it is full of "earth Qi" or healing energy. This nurturing quality is lost when the herb is stored for months or years, or when the herb is subjected to extensive processing, especially if harsh industrial solvents are used.

Dandelion, garlic, rosemary, and thyme are just some of the fresh herbs that lend themselves to easy use. Dandelion leaf is a potent diuretic and helps push excess water out of the body; in French, its name translates to "pee-a-bed". Rosemary, thyme, and garlic are used as seasonings in many dishes, and increasing their use gives one more access to their digestive, antimicrobial, and cardiovascular support actions.

Fresh lemon balm, rubbed on the skin, keeps insects away. Use the tender top leaves, which contain the most oil. Pinching these back also encourages the plant to branch out and become full.

Feverfew leaves, eaten fresh, guard against migraine, although they are quite bitter and many prefer to disguise them in other foods. It's very gratifying to see feverfew at work. The father of a friend of mine suffered from migraine headaches throughout his adult life. At last he agreed to try feverfew. He ate one leaf twice daily from the plant in his garden, but after three months experienced no change. At that point, his doctor suggested he give up this "silliness" and try a new migraine medication, but the father persisted with the feverfew. After five months, the intensity and frequency of his headaches were reduced, and after seven months he was free of migraine for the first time in many years. That was two years ago, and he remains headache-free today.

MAKING HERBAL MEDICINES TASTE GOOD

It's been decades since Mary Poppins declared that "a spoonful of sugar helps the medicine go down", but my years of creating medicinal formulations have proved the truth of her statement. The most important basic rule for medicinal formulations is this: They must have appeal.

If a preparation tastes bad—or, in the case of a topical preparation, smells or looks bad—it won't be used. Of course, tastes differ, but a good liquid product for internal consumption should have an inviting taste and smell. A good external product should have a consistent texture and a fresh, healthful scent.

Some herbal teas and decoctions, despite their curative powers, taste odd or downright awful. While one might develop tolerance to the taste of many, others require additions to become palatable. If a recipe in this chapter doesn't seem enticing to you as you're making it, consider adding more pleasant-tasting herbs such as licorice, anise, or cinnamon to the brew. Orange or grapefruit peel also add flavor. Stevia is a powerful herbal sweetener that helps take the edge off even bitter teas, and honey combines well, too.

ESSENTIAL OILS TO TRY

These essential oils are useful for their inviting aromas as well as their healing properties.

Camphor stimulates the nerves, increases blood circulation, and relieves pain. It's an active ingredient of Vick's Vaporub. Use externally only.

Clove should be used in small amounts. When used in tea or sprinkled liberally on food, it is a pain reliever.

Eucalyptus oil is a strong antiseptic, and it's used in cough and throat products for its decongestant properties.

Lavender has an old-fashioned, familiar smell that lifts the spirits. It's one of the best all-around oils for body products, although it can be used for flavoring, too.

Orange, like *lemon*, is nicely scented and can be used internally or externally.

Peppermint has a cool, refreshing scent and taste, but a little goes a long way. Use this oil to ease intestinal cramps and gas pains or soothe an inflamed throat or a cough.

Rosemary oil is strongly antiseptic and stimulating to the nervous system. Include it in products that relieve the pain of chapped lips or abraded skin.

Sage has a strong, earthy smell and is one of the most antiseptic oils. It can be irritating; use a small amount.

Tea tree's nice woodsy scent makes it a natural for external preparations designed for men. It is strongly antibacterial and antifungal without being too irritating, but used undiluted it can cause peeling skin.

Thyme is strongly antibacterial and warming. When used in concentrated form, it can be very irritating; it is best used externally only.

Essential Additives

Small amounts of essential oils can be used to improve the taste, smell, and medicinal qualities of herbal preparations. This requires a careful hand, for a few drops are usually enough.

These oils are extremely concentrated and should never be taken internally without professional advice. Many are toxic. Some even cause problems when used externally; for example, thyme essential oil is extremely irritating to the skin. On the other hand, used carefully in the recommended small quantities, they are a quick and easy way to add flavors, scents, and medicinal properties to preparations.

The Recipes

The first recipes given here are model recipes, simple single-herb combinations that allow the substitution of other herbs. These recipes serve as models for your information and exploration; using the same measurements of herb and liquid, you may substitute herbs freely using these basic recipes.

For example, the model recipe for infusion specifies chamomile, but other herbs can be substituted with good results. Just use the same amount of dried or fresh herb and the same amount of water. The model recipe for infused oil uses calendula; if you want arnica oil instead, use an identical amount of that herb. The Basic Dried Tea recipe is similar.

The model tincture recipe is different because each herb requires a different solvent, although the recipe calls for 3 ounces of dried herb for each 16 ounces of solvent. Find that herb's solvent in Table 1, beginning on page 113, and mix it up; then start the recipe.

The following recipes in this chapter are more complex combinations of herbs that I've used in my practice with excellent results.

ABOUT HERBAL TEAS

Teas, often called infusions and decoctions, are one of the oldest and easiest ways to take herbal medicines. Infusions gently extract the healing compounds from fragile leaves and flowers; decoctions use more heat and time to reap the medicine from woody parts of plants.

Basic Infusion: Chamomile Tea

Chamomile flower tea is a traditional remedy to help relax the bowels and relieve cramps, irritability, and inflammation. Mothers all over the world use chamomile tea to relieve their babies' painful colic.

3 tablespoons (45 ml) dried
chamomile flowers
OR 5 (75 ml) tablespoons fresh
3 cups water (711 ml)

Bring water to a boil and remove from heat. Add flowers, cover, and steep for 15 to 20 minutes. When cool, store in the refrigerator. Drink 1 cup (237 ml), warmed, two to three times a day, preferably away from meal times.

WARM-WATER INFUSIONS

These herbs require only infusion in warm water to release their healing qualities. Place them in a clean, covered container filled with room-temperature water for up to 8 hours, strain, and drink.

Catnip helps babies with colic and everyone else, too, who has digestive upset.

Chamomile calms the nerves and soothes the digestive system; it's good after dinner or before bed.

Feverfew, taken regularly, helps protect against migraine headaches.

Hawthorn flowering tops make a pleasant-tasting and mildly relaxing tea.

Lavender tea is fragrant and calming; it eases digestion.

Lemon balm, an antioxidant herb, smells and tastes lemony and lifts the spirit.

Lemon verbena tea, taken daily, allays insomnia and improves digestive functions.

Marshmallow root can help if you suspect a bladder infection; chop the herb fine and steep overnight. Drink the liquid in the morning.

Mugwort tea promotes good fat digestion and relieves menstrual pain when sipped as needed.

Peppermint tea soothes an upset stomach.

Red clover tea is diuretic and cleanses the blood.

Red raspberry leaves make an excellent gentle tonic for use during pregnancy.

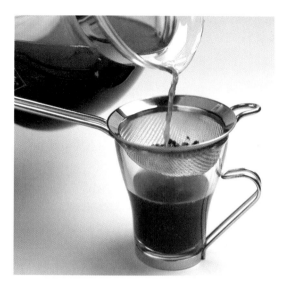

Basic Decoction: Yellow Dock Root and Licorice

Yellow dock is an excellent cleansing herb, especially when combined with licorice. It can also be used for short-term constipation. Licorice reduces inflammation and has a soothing effect on the digestive system. Its sweet taste improves the palatability of the tea. This recipe accommodates most roots, barks, and other woody plant materials. Vary the amount of herb according to your taste and need.

2 tablespoons (30 ml) dried yellow dock root
2 tablespoons (30 ml) licorice root
1 ½ cup (355 ml) water

Grind the roots in a blender or food processor. Place roots in cold water in a saucepan. Heat and simmer, uncovered, until liquid is reduced about a third. Strain to remove herb. Store liquid in refrigerator. Drink half a cup (118 ml) three or four times daily.

ABOUT INFUSED OILS

Herbal infused oils are made by grinding coarsely the fresh or dried herbs and blending them into oil. The mixture steeps for about two or three weeks and should be stirred or shaken daily. After careful filtering to remove the herb, the finished oil can be bottled and refrigerated.

In selecting an oil for infusing, choose a light, high-quality one. Olive oil is my favorite; it does not spoil easily and can be used both internally and externally. I prefer the cold-pressed extra-virgin oil that comes from the first pressing of the olives and has never been heated. You may use other oils as you desire.

Quick Plantain Infused Oil

Here's a quick way to make herbal infused oil; the method can be used with any herb. This plantain oil is helpful for wounds, hemorrhoids, and sores; it encourages the healing of damaged tissue.

2 cups fresh plantain leaves (474 ml)
2 cups oil (474 ml)

In a blender, process the leaves and oil until smooth. Place the mixture in a crock pot turned to low, or about 100 degrees Fahrenheit (37° C.). Cover. To prevent spoilage, keep herb submerged in oil at all times; add more oil if necessary. Stir daily for five to seven days. Let the oil cool and strain, pressing the oil from the herb. Bottle and store in the refrigerator.

Calendula Infused Oil

Calendula infused oil is great for burns, scrapes, rashes, itchy skin, and other skin trauma. It can form the base for calendula salves and creams.

1 ½ cup dried calendula flowers (355 ml)
2 cups oil (474 ml)

In a blender, process the flowers and oil until smooth. Pour the mixture into a quart jar or other container, cover, and put in a warm place out of the direct sunlight. Shake the jar vigorously every day for two to three weeks. The herb must be submerged in the oil at all times to prevent mold and fungus. *If necessary, add more oil.* Using a fine strainer or cloth, filter the herb out of the oil, pressing as much oil out as possible. Bottle the oil for use and refrigerate.

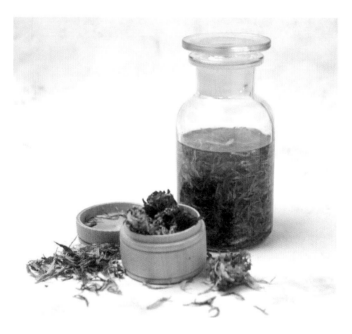

ABOUT TINCTURES

Tinctures are popular because they're concentrated and convenient to use. A full dose is only a few droppersful in a cup of water several times per day. Tinctures are best prepared with single herbs. Mix tinctures if you wish, but make each individually. Freshly shade-dried herbs usually give the best results. This recipe can be used to make glycerites or vinegars as well by substituting those ingredients for the solvent. Double or triple the recipe as desired. The recipe here is for echinacea tincture, but any herb can be substituted.

Echinacea Tincture

6 tablespoons (3 ounces or 90 ml) echinacea dried root, chopped
2 cup (16 ounces or 474 ml) solvent as indicated in Table 1, page 113

Mix the solvent indicated in Table 1 for the desired herb. Echinacea dried root, for instance, requires a solvent of alcohol:water of 60/40, or 9.5 ounces (284 ml) grain alcohol combined with 6.5 ounces (190 ml) distilled water.

In a clean, lidded glass jar, combine herb and solvent. Cover the jar and store in a dark place, shaking daily for two to three weeks. Do not allow the herb to float above the level of the alcohol or the tincture will spoil; add more alcohol if necessary.

When the tincture is finished, filter the mixture Squeeze out the last drops of liquid from the herbs, preferably with a sturdy herb press. Discard the herb and pour the tincture into labeled amber bottles. Shelf life for alcohol tinctures is up to three years.

HEALING TEA BLENDS

Three-Seed Tea

This delicious tea is a favorite among many of my patients for preventing gas after meals.

2 teaspoons cumin seed (10 ml)
2 teaspoons fennel seed (10 ml)
2 teaspoons caraway seed (10 ml)
1 teaspoon orange peel, chopped (5 ml)
½ teaspoon licorice root, chopped (2.5 ml)
½ teaspoon peppermint (2.5 ml)
3 cups water (711 ml)

Place seeds, orange peel, and licorice root in water. Simmer in covered pot for 20 minutes. Remove from heat, add peppermint, and let steep, covered, for 15 minutes. Strain and discard herbs. Drink 1 cup (237 ml) up to three times a day. Store cold.

Sleep Deep Tea

This is a blend of pleasant herbs to help relax body and mind and promote a deep, refreshing sleep.

2 teaspoons chamomile flowers (10 ml)
2 teaspoons passion flower (10 ml)
1 teaspoon St. John's wort (5 ml)
1 teaspoon lemon balm (5 ml)
1 teaspoon valerian root (5 ml)

1 teaspoon hops flowers (5 ml)
1 teaspoon catnip herb (5 ml)
½ teaspoon stevia for sweetness (2.5 ml)
3 cups water (711 ml)

Infuse the herbs in freshly boiled water in a covered pot for 20 minutes. Strain out herb and discard. Drink one or two cups (up to 474 ml) as desired. Store tea in the refrigerator.

Cold and Flu Brew

This classic blend is comforting and healing during the misery of a cold or flu. It helps remove heat and toxins from the body, fights the viral infection, and acts as a decongestant.

2 ¼ teaspoons echinacea leaf (11 ml)
2 ¼ teaspoons elder flowers (11 ml)
2 ¼ teaspoons yarrow flowers and leaf (11 ml)
1 ¾ teaspoons peppermint (9 ml)
¼ teaspoon stevia (optional) (1.25 ml)
3 cups water (711 ml)

Place all herbs except peppermint in water and simmer, covered, for 10 to 15 minutes. Remove from heat, add peppermint, and steep, covered, for 10 minutes. Strain herb and discard. Drink up to three cups tea daily as needed. Store tea in the refrigerator.

Cleansing Tea

This fantastic tea contains cleansing, liver stimulating, cooling, and soothing herbs to reduce inflammation or irritation in the entire digestive tract, along with giving the system a good cleanse. It tastes great, too!

2 ¼ teaspoons fennel seed (11 ml)
2 ¼ teaspoons fenugreek seed (11 ml)
2 ¼ teaspoons flax seed (11 ml)
heaping ¼ teaspoon fresh ginger root,
finely chopped (1.5 ml)
heaping ¼ teaspoon dried licorice root, (1.5 ml)
heaping ¼ teaspoon teaspoons peppermint (1.5 ml)
3 cups water (711 ml)

Add all ingredients except peppermint to water. Simmer, covered, for 20 minutes. Add peppermint and steep, covered, for ten minutes. Strain; discard herbs. Drink 1 cup (237 ml) three times a day as desired. Store tea in the refrigerator.

Calming After-Dinner Tea

A cup or two of this relaxing and delicious tea is the perfect ending to a satisfying meal.

1 tablespoon linden (15 ml)
2 teaspoons lemon balm (10 ml)
2 teaspoons lemon chamomile flowers (10 ml)
1 ½ teaspoons fennel seed (7.5 ml)
1 teaspoon oatstraw (5 ml)
½ teaspoon stevia (optional) (2.5 ml)
3 cups water (711 ml)

Infuse the herbs in freshly boiled water in a covered pot for 20 minutes. Strain out herb and discard. Drink 1 or 2 cups as desired. Store cold.

Stress-Buster Tea

This tea supports the adrenal glands and helps counteract the harmful effects of stress.

1 tablespoon eleuthero root (Siberian ginseng) (15 ml)
2 teaspoons linden flowers (10 ml)
2 teaspoons oatstraw (10 ml)
1 teaspoon kava kava root (5 ml)
1 teaspoon orange peel (5 ml)
¼ teaspoon stevia herb (or to taste for sweetness) (1.25 ml)
3 cups water (711 ml)

Simmer in a covered pan or pot for 10 minutes, steep for about 15 minutes, strain and drink as needed, up to 5 cups (1180 ml) a day.

Immune-Support Tea

This decoction strengthens natural immunity

2 ¼ teaspoons ligustrum (11 ml)
2 ¼ teaspoons gynostemma (optional) (11 ml)
1 ⅛ teaspoon astragalus root (5.5 ml)
1 ⅛ teaspoon reishi mushrooms (5.5 ml)
1 ⅛ teaspoon shiitake mushrooms (5.5 ml)
¾ teaspoon licorice root (3 ml)
5 cups water (1180 ml)

Grind all herbs coarsely. Add all herbs except gynostemma to the pot and simmer, uncovered, for 45 minutes or until liquid is reduced by one fourth. Remove from heat, add gynostemma, cover, and steep for 15 minutes. Strain; discard herbs. Drink 1 cup (237 ml) three times a day as needed. Store cold.

Moon-Cycle Tea

This herbal blend for premenstrual syndrome and regulating menstrual irregularity balances the hormones, cools the liver, eases cramps and pain, and helps reduce inflammation. The tea is most effective if drunk beginning at ovulation—the center of the cycle—through the end of the menstrual period.

1 tablespoon burdock root (15 ml)
2 teaspoons blue cohosh (10 ml)
1 teaspoon black cohosh (5 ml)
1 teaspoon wild yam root (5 ml)
1 teaspoon cramp bark (5 ml)
1 teaspoon orange peel (5 ml)
1 teaspoon licorice root (5 ml)
3 ⅓ cups water (790 ml)

Place herbs in water and simmer uncovered for 30 minutes. Cover and let steep for 10 minutes. Strain; discard herbs. Drink ½ to 1 cup (up to 237 ml) three times daily as needed.

Menopause Tea

The herbs in this tea have a mild estrogenic effect, regulate all the female hormones, move and build the blood, and have a general strengthening effect on the female organs.

2 teaspoons stinging nettles (10 ml)
1 teaspoon vitex berries (5 ml)
1 teaspoon black cohosh root (5 ml)
1 teaspoon lavender flowers (5 ml)

1 teaspoon dong quai root (5 ml)
1 teaspoon fennel seed (5 ml)
1 teaspoon fenugreek seed (5 ml)
1 teaspoon licorice root or stevia, or to taste (5 ml)
3 cups water (711 ml)

Mince roots and berries. Simmer all ingredients in a covered pot for 15 minutes. Remove from heat and let steep, covered, for about 15 minutes. Strain and drink as needed, up to 3 cups (711 ml) a day. This tea can be used at room temperature.

Winter Inhalation

This traditional herbal steam helps open sinuses, discourages bacterial and viral growth, and reduces pain and inflammation.

4 teaspoons eucalyptus leaves (20 ml)
1 tablespoon peppermint (15 ml)
1 tablespoon thyme (15 ml)
3 cups water (711 ml)

Simmer the herb blend in a covered pot for 5 to 10 minutes. Remove from heat and uncover. Drape a large towel over your head and the pot, forming a steam-filled tent, and inhale the medicated steam deeply for five minutes or so. Repeat several times daily as needed. *Caution:* Do not place your face too close to the pot or burns may result.

Enhance the inhalation by adding six or seven drops of essential oil to the brew for increased potency. For this inhalation, oils of eucalyptus, peppermint, and thyme are appropriate; add one or more as desired. Do not use enhanced inhalations more than two or three times a day, however. The essential oils can cause dizziness and light-headedness. If redness of the mucous membranes develops, discontinue.

Talking Herbs:
A Soothing Throat Gargle

This gargle soothes throats that are sore from overuse, a condition experienced by anyone who becomes hoarse after using the voice excessively.

2 $^1/_2$ tablespoons echinacea leaf (37 ml)
2 tablespoons lemon balm (30 ml)
2 tablespoons witch hazel (30 ml)
1 $^1/_2$ tablespoons sage leaf (23 ml)
1 $^1/_2$ tablespoons usnea* (if available) (23 ml)
1 $^1/_2$ teaspoons licorice root part (7.5 ml)
5 cups water (1180 ml)

Simmer the herbs in water for 15 minutes, covered. Remove from heat and steep for 10 minutes. Strain out herb and discard; store in the refrigerator. Gargle ¼ cup of the warm or at least room-temperature tea four or five times a day; if swallowed, no harm will result. For portability, carry a little dropper bottle; 3 or 4 droppersful gargled for 30 seconds is a quick fix.

* Any of the *Usnea* species—lichens, lungwort *(Lobaria oregana* or *L. pulmonaria)*, or Iceland moss *(Centraria islandica)* can be used interchangeably. All have soothing, expectorant, and antibacterial actions.

DRIED TEAS

While some of my patients enjoy making herbal teas, others don't have the time to prepare and enjoy these healthful beverages. So I keep on hand a large selection of dried teas—teas that have been concentrated and then dried in the fruit-leather trays of a food dehydrator.

Dried teas are very concentrated. One-half teaspoon of a powdered dried tea actually contains all the active and desirable constituents of up to five teaspoons of the herb. These preparations are potent, convenient, and effective ways of using tonic herbs for greater health and increased energy. They work slowly, but over time often bring dramatic results.

Basic Dried Tea:
Stinging Nettles and Horsetail

Begin making this tea by putting on rubber gloves if using fresh stinging nettles.

4 cups stinging nettle (950 ml)
4 cups horsetail (950 ml)
10 cups water (2370 ml)

Simmer uncovered for two to four hours or until a dark, strong tea is created. Let cool until warm.

Remove half of the boiled herbs and press or squeeze them as dry as possible, catching the liquid to return to the pot. Discard the spent herbs. Again simmer the tea until the water level is reduced by another three-fourths. Let cool until warm. In a blender, process this strong mixture until creamy. If the mix seems watery, simmer it again until it is thicker.

Pour this "batter" into the fruit-leather trays of a food dehydrator set at 100 to 120 degrees Fahrenheit (37°C.). Dry the mix completely.

The tea will be a thin, dry solid that is easily broken or powdered in a blender. Store the wafer, broken up or powdered, in an amber glass jar away from direct sunlight.

Tips: If you wish, tinctures of herbs such as orange peel, ginger, or echinacea can be stirred into the cooled mix as it dries, either to add medicinal effects or better taste. Tinctures of herbs such as valerian that contain delicate essential oils and other sensitive compounds remain effective when added in this way.

Try stirring in finely powdered licorice root, eleuthero powder, and other herb powders into the tea concentrate before drying to prevent sticking to the trays and give the final product more body.

Dosage: Eat a piece the size of a quarter up to a silver dollar two or three times daily, or make an instant tea by adding ½ to 1 teaspoon (5ml) of the wafer or powder to warm or hot water. If the blend upsets your stomach, drink it just before mealtimes. If the tea is powdered and placed into 00-size gelatin capsules, a daily dose is two or three capsules (½ gram), two or three times daily with meals.

Vitamineral Blend Dried Tea

This dried-tea recipe uses herbs that are storehouses of easily assimilated vitamins and minerals. Take this blend regularly to strengthen hair, skin, nails, bones, and connective tissue. Use rubber gloves while handling the stinging nettles.

4 cups stinging nettle (950 ml)
3 cups horsetail (711 ml)
3 cups plantain (711 ml)
Licorice (optional) small amount
3 quarts water (3 liters)

Simmer uncovered for two to four hours or until a dark, strong tea is formed. Let cool until warm. Remove half of the boiled herbs and press or squeeze them dry, catching the liquid to return to the pot. Discard the spent herbs. Simmer the tea again until the water level is reduced by another three-fourths. Allow to cool.

In a blender, process the mixture of tea and herb until creamy. If the mix seems watery, simmer it again until it is thicker.

Pour this "batter" into the fruit-leather trays of a food dehydrator set at 100 to 120 degrees Fahrenheit (37°C.). Dry the mix completely. To enhance assimilation, tinctures of herbs such as orange peel or ginger can be stirred into the cooled mix as it dries.

The tea will be a thin, dry solid that is easily broken or powdered in a blender. Store in an amber glass jar away from direct sunlight. Follow the dosage directions for the Basic Dried Tea.

Strengthen-the-Middle Dried Tea

This recipe has helped many people regain digestive strength and remove excess water from the body.

2 cups ginger root, (474 ml)
¾ cup ginseng, red Korean or Chinese (178 ml)
½ cup poria (also called fu ling) (118 ml)
1 cup orange peel (237 ml)
3 quarts water (3 liters)
2 cups (474 ml) astragalus root
½ cup (118 ml) eleuthero powder
1 ounce tincture of artichoke leaf (30 ml)

Simmer first five ingredients uncovered for two to four hours or until a dark, strong tea is formed. Let cool until warm. Remove half of the boiled herbs and press or squeeze them dry, catching the liquid to return to the pot. Discard the spent herbs.

Simmer the tea again until the water level is reduced by another three-fourths. Allow to cool. In a blender, process the mixture of tea and herb until creamy. The mix should be a bit watery.

When the batter is almost cool, add tincture and eleuthero powder; stir. Spread the concentrate on the fruit-leather trays of a food dehydrator and dry at 100 to 120 degrees Fahrenheit (37°C.). Break up the dried blend or powder it and store away from heat and light. Follow the dosage directions for the Basic Dried Tea.

BATH TEAS

A good warm bath at the end of a busy day—at any time, in fact—can be a healing as well as a pleasing experience. Enhance warm water's natural relaxing qualities with a strong herbal tea poured directly into the bath. Some herbal benefits will be absorbed effortlessly through the skin. Others, such as volatile oils, will rise from the surface of the water with the steam.

! *Caution: Bath teas are much stronger than teas for drinking, and they should not be taken internally. Label these teas clearly, and store away from the kitchen.*

Bedtime Bath Tea

This bath tea's wonderful fragrance relaxes the spirit, and its healing substances soften the skin. It helps children calm down in the evening.

For a single bath:

3 tablespoons chamomile flowers (45 ml)
3 tablespoons lemon balm (45 ml)
2 tablespoons lavender flowers (30 ml)
2 tablespoons linden flowers (30 ml)
6 cups water (1422 ml)
Several drops essential oil such as lavender, grapefruit, or cedar (optional)

Simmer the herbs in water for five minutes, covered, and let steep for 20 minutes. If desired, strain the herbs from the tea and discard. Add essential oil and shake well. Add the tea to a warm bath and enjoy.

Healthy Skin Bath Tea

These herbs are especially soothing during gardening season, when mosquito bites, scratches and scrapes, and a little sunburn are likely.

For a single bath:
1 tablespoon calendula flowers (15 ml)
1 tablespoon plantain leaves (15 ml)
1 tablespoon gotu kola (15 ml)
1 tablespoon lavender flowers (15 ml)
1 tablespoon echinacea leaves (15 ml)
1 tablespoon ginger root (15 ml)
2 cups water (474 ml)

Place the herbs in a covered pot and simmer for 30 minutes. Strain out and discard herbs if desired. Add the tea to a warm bath and enjoy.

Colds and Flu Bath Tea

Mix a cup of each of these dried herbs together in the early autumn and store in an airtight container away from heat and light. All winter, you'll have this comforting blend ready to steep when illness threatens. This bath tea combines herbs that cause sweating, support the immune system, and relieve sore muscles. Omit the ginger if you or family members tend to have fevers during illness.

For a single bath:
1 tablespoon wintergreen leaves (15 ml)
1 tablespoon echinacea leaves (15 ml)
1 tablespoon ginger root, chopped or grated fine (15 ml)

1 tablespoon yarrow flowers and leaves (15 ml)
1 tablespoon eucalyptus leaves (15 ml)
2 cups water (474 ml)
Or, if making in quantity: ⅓ cup of the herb blend and 5
to 6 cups (up to 1416 ml) of water.

Simmer, covered, for 30 minutes. Strain out and discard herbs if desired. Add the tea to a hot, steamy bath and enjoy. For a stronger, therapeutic bath, double or triple the recipe.

COMPRESS TEAS

Compresses are another way to use herbal teas for healing wounds, rashes, and skin infections. Soak a clean linen, cotton, or gauze cloth in strong tea, fold it to size, and apply it to the affected area. A cool compress soothes itching or burning pain, but a warm compress is better for aches and infections. Top a

---

SOOTHING COMPRESSES FOR EVERYDAY USE

Calendula tea in a warm compress helps heal wounds and varicose ulcers.

Chamomile tea soothes sunburn or rash with a cool compress.

Lemon balm is an antiviral; use cool compress to apply it to chickenpox and other herpes outbreaks.

Rosemary in a warm compress helps relieve the pain of arthritis or sore muscles.

Thyme in a warm compress of strong tea will prevent or relieve surface infections.

---

warm compress with a hot water bottle to maintain the temperature; similarly, an ice pack wrapped in a towel will keep a cold compress chilled.

Eye-Love-Herbs Compress Tea

This traditional formula is often recommended by herbalists to soothe red, irritated eyes and reduce the inflammation and infection of pinkeye and styes.

1 teaspoon goldenseal rhizome (5 ml)
1 tablespoon eyebright herb (15 ml)
½ cup water (118 ml)

Simmer herbs in a covered pot for 10 minutes. Remove from heat and let herbs steep for 15 minutes. Strain out the herb and discard. Soak a sterile cotton pad in the tea and cover the infected eye. Tape in

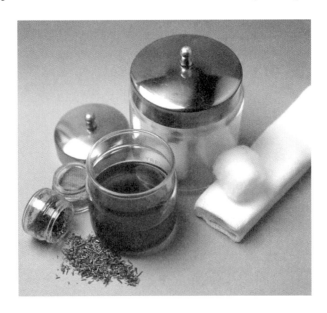

place; remoisten as needed. Change two or three times a day; leave on overnight. Alternately, use the cool tea in an eye cup two or three times a day.

Rash Compress Tea

The herbs in this formula are astringent, soothing, and healing. Use this compress for poison ivy and oak, hives, blackheads, and acne that does not come to a head for draining.

⅞ cup calendula flowers (207 ml)
⅝ cup witch hazel bark (148 ml)
½ cup gotu kola leaves (118 ml)
½ cup white oak bark (118 ml)
10 cups water (2360 ml)

Grind the herbs and simmer in water, covered, for about 20 minutes. Let cool and wrap about ¼ cup (59 ml) or more of the wet herbs in a muslin or other porous cloth.

Apply the herbs to the affected area for 10 to 15 minutes. Resoak the herbs in the tea and apply again; repeat one more time. Repeat for two or three sessions daily, as needed.

For hot, itchy rashes, blend several drops of peppermint oil into the compress herbs before applying them to the skin.

Between compress sessions, apply to the skin some St. John's wort infused oil to which a few drops of peppermint oil have been added. Calendula oil or cream or aloe vera gel may be used as well.

Wound and Acne Compress Tea

These herbs have a long history of successful use in expediting wound healing by activating the healing response as well as reducing soreness, inflammation, and pain. Applied externally, the herbs are effective against acne, boils, cuts, bites, stings, and infection.

1 cup plantain leaves (237 ml)
½ cup yarrow flowers and leaves (118 ml)
¼ cup Oregon grape root (60 ml)
2 cups water (474 ml)

Simmer the herbs uncovered for 20 minutes, remove from heat, cover and steep for 15 minutes. Strain out the herb and place it in a muslin or other porous cloth and apply to skin trauma. Resoak the herbs in the tea and reapply two or three times. Repeat two or three times per day until skin is healed.

Herbal Glycerites

Glycerites are another way to take herbs—a way that is gaining in popularity. If you like to taste your herbs, yet are tired of swallowing handfuls of pills and don't want to consume alcohol, then herbal glycerites might be just right for you. Some parents also prefer glycerites for administering herbs to children.

Herbal glycerites can be made in two ways. The dried or fresh herbs can be blended with pure vegetable glycerin until smooth, just as you would make an alcohol tincture. Shake the mixture every day for two weeks, and then press or squeeze out the finished liquid. Filter it if a clear finished product is desired. A second way to make glycerites is to carefully and slowly evaporate the alcohol from a tincture over an electric burner, then add an amount of glycerin equal to the original amount of alcohol.

Sweet-smelling essential oils can be added to a glycerite to enhance the flavor and aroma. Tangerine, orange, lemon, and mint oils are especially popular.

Echinacea-Orange Glycerite

1 ½ ounce dried echinacea flowers and leaves (45 ml)
8 ounces pure vegetable glycerin (237 ml)
1 ounce honey (30 ml)
20-30 drops essential oil (orange, tangerine, or cinnamon)

Put herb and glycerin in a blender and whirl until smooth. Pour contents into a canning jar or other suitable container. Keep in a warm place and shake daily for 2 to 3 weeks.

Pour the contents of the jar into a muslin bag. Squeeze out the liquid and discard the spent herbs. If desired, add honey for sweetness and essential oil for flavor. Mix well. Put into small amber bottles with droppers.

The dose is 1 to 3 droppersful of the glycerite 3 to 4 times daily for a week to ten days, away from meal times. This glycerite helps stave off colds or flu. If illness has set in, increase the dose to 1 to 3 droppersful every few hours for about a week. For children, use half this dose, more or less depending on the child's age and weight.

Herbal Syrups

Herbal sweets are favored by kids of all ages. Any herbal tea can be concentrated and added to a sweet base for a syrup. Because this process concentrates the herb's active constituents, the remedy produced is very effective.

After making syrup, bottle it, label it, and store it in the refrigerator. If no preservatives are added, it will probably last up to two or three weeks. Adding essential oils will increase its refrigerated shelf life a week or two more. If it's impractical to store the syrup in the refrigerator, add 25 percent grain alcohol or 75 percent vegetable glycerin. This comes in handy if you are traveling.

Horehound and Orange Cough Syrup

1 ½ teaspoons horehound leaf (8 ml)
1 ½ teaspoons echinacea root (8 ml)
¾ teaspoons sage leaf (4 ml)
1 ½ teaspoons orange peel (8 ml)
¾ teaspoons licorice root (4 ml)
1 ½ teaspoons wild cherry bark (8 ml)
1 ½ teaspoons thyme (8 ml)
4 cups water (948 ml)
1 ¼ cups honey (295 ml)
¾ cup barley malt (178 ml)
7 drops orange essential oil
3 drops peppermint essential oil

Grind herbs and simmer in water for 10 minutes; steep 20 minutes. Return to heat and cook uncovered until one quarter of the original amount is left. Add honey, barley malt, and essential oils; stir well, bottle, and store.

Variations. While the syrup is still warm, add a total of 10 drops of one or two essential oils and mix thoroughly.

Thyme is strongly antibacterial but harsh, so use only 5 to 10 drops per cup of syrup.

Eucalyptus is antibacterial, decongestant, and moderately harsh; use 5 to 15 drops per cup of syrup.

Peppermint and *orange* cool the throat, calm coughs, and taste good, too.

Cinnamon is warming and imparts a familiar flavor to the syrup.

Stevia is a sweetener; a little bit goes a long way.

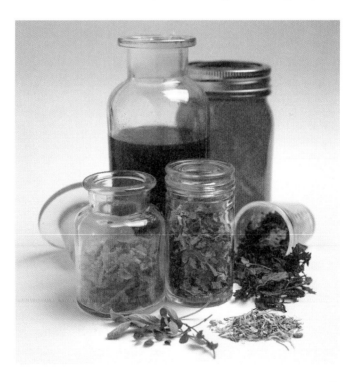

TOPICAL MEDICINES

Applying healing herbs to the skin can stop bleeding, protect against infection, and ease pain. The skin also absorbs some constituents, so certain herbs applied to the skin can stimulate internal organs or blood circulation, thus encouraging healing.

POULTICES AND PLASTERS

Poultices are made by adding hot water to dried, powdered herbs or fresh, coarsely ground herbs and placing the herb directly on the affected area. The herbs may be covered with gauze and taped in place. They can be kept warm with a hot water bottle or heating pad and are preferably left on overnight or for a few hours.

Plasters are oily or waxy mixtures blended with herbs and applied to the chest area or abdomen to stimulate the internal organs. In past times, the mixture was spread onto a cloth and rolled tightly for storage, then unrolled and applied when needed.

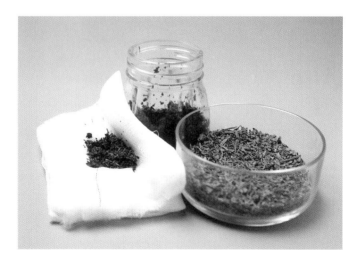

Plantain Poultice

This classic herbal preparation can be applied to burns, cuts, scrapes, or other injuries to reduce inflammation, prevent infection, and speed healing.

½ cup (118 ml) dried plantain leaves or
a handful of fresh ones
Boiling water

Place about ¼ cup (59 ml) hot water in blender jar and add plantain. Begin blending and slowly add water until the mixture becomes thick enough to spread. It should not be watery; the mucilage in the herb will form a thick, gooey paste. If you don't have access to fresh plantain leaves—I highly recommend growing them in your garden—dried leaf can be purchased from an herb supplier.

Onion Poultice

This poultice eases coughs, bronchitis, and pneumonia. It's safe for children—pick out a good story to read while the poultice is doing its work.

1 large onion, chopped coarsely
3 tablespoons flax seed (45 ml)
2 tablespoons olive oil (30 ml)

Place ingredients in a frying pan and sauté until the onions are translucent. Wrap the onions and flax seed in cheesecloth and apply to the chest while as warm as possible. Cover with a hot water bottle and a towel. Leave on for 20 to 30 minutes.

Mustard Plaster

This plaster stimulates the flow and release of mucus from the lungs and bronchial area and promotes blood flow and healing. Use one when colds or flu cause chest congestion.

⅓ cup mustard seed, finely ground (79 ml)
Olive oil
Beeswax, grated

Place a tablespoon or two of oil into the blender jar and add ground mustard. Blend, slowly adding enough olive oil to make a thick liquid. Pour oil into a pan and heat gently, just hot enough to melt beeswax. Slowly add grated beeswax, testing for hardness by dipping out a metal spoonful and dipping the bowl of the spoon in ice water. This salve should be somewhat harder (more waxy) than a regular salve.

While the preparation is warm and spreadable, apply evenly to a linen or cotton cloth about 5" by 5" or another suitable size. Let the plaster harden before using; it can be stored in the refrigerator in a plastic bag for future use if desired.

When it is needed, take the plaster out of the refrigerator and let it warm to room temperature. Place it mustard-side down on the chest, over the lungs. After 10 or 15 minutes, the area should start turning red and the patient will feel the heat of the mustard. Leave the plaster on for another 10 to 15 minutes until the area is thoroughly warmed and stimulated. The plaster can be applied daily for two to five days until the chest is loosened up and breathing is free.

! *Don't leave on longer than 30 to 40 minutes or deep burns can result! Check every 5 to 10 minutes to see if the area is red and hot. Never let the patient fall asleep while using the plaster.*

Earache Oil

This classic formula is a must for every family medicine chest and first-aid kit. It combines the bacteriostatic properties of mullein flowers with the antibacterial action of garlic to prevent and ease earaches, wax buildup, and irritation.

1 tablespoon fresh garlic clove (15 ml)
2 tablespoons fresh or dried mullein flower (30 ml)
½ cup olive or almond oil to cover (118 ml)

Crush garlic well and break up mullein flower; place herbs into blender jar. Cover with oil and blend well. Pour the mixture into a clean, clear jar and store away from heat and light. Shake the jar daily. To prevent spoilage, keep herb submerged in oil at all times; add more oil if necessary. After two weeks, strain the herb from the oil and discard. Store oil in the refrigerator.

To use, put two or three drops of the oil into the ear. Tilt the head so the oil flows easily down the ear canal. Massage the back of the ear several times to aid in dispersing the oil throughout the ear canal.

! *Whenever a child has an ear infection, consult a qualified healthcare practitioner before treating it at home. Do the same for an adult with a severe ear infection.*

St. John's Wort Infused Oil

St. John's wort infused oil helps heal damaged nerves as well as other tissues. Conscientious, regular massage of the injured area with the oil can bring astonishing healing, even to old injuries. Taken internally, this oil helps heal stomach ulcers.

1 ½ cups dried St. John's wort (355 ml)
2 cups oil (474 ml)

In a blender, process the herb and oil until smooth. Pour the mixture into a clear glass jar and cover. This oil should become bright red as it develops; if it does not, place the jar on a sunny window sill where sunlight can act on it. To prevent spoilage, keep herb submerged in oil at all times; add more oil if necessary. Shake the jar vigorously every day for two to three weeks. Filter the herb from the oil, pressing as much oil out as possible. Bottle the oil and refrigerate.

Aches 'n Pains Oil

Use this effective combination of herbal oils for a healing rub for sore and strained muscles as well as sprains.

4 teaspoons St. John's wort infused oil (20 ml)
2 teaspoons arnica infused oil (10 ml)
10 drops wintergreen essential oil

Make each herbal infused oil separately using either the two-week or crock-pot method. Mix the oils with essential oil and shake well. Apply to sore muscles, joints, tendons, and ligaments, but avoid broken skin. Store in the refrigerator. If desired, 10 drops of eucalyptus essential oil may be substituted for the wintergreen essential oil.

! *This product is toxic! Do not take this oil internally, and discontinue use if you notice skin redness or irritation.*

ENHANCING INFUSED OILS

Expand the usefulness of herbal infused oils by adding small quantities of essential oils. Five to ten drops of essential oil in ¼ cup (59 ml) of infused oil is sufficient, but do not take the enhanced oil internally. Here are some suggestions for adding essential oils to infused oils:

Lavender essential oil is effective against tension and headache when rubbed into the temples and neck. Add to chamomile infused oil to treat eczema.

Wintergreen essential oil soothes muscle aches resulting from arthritis or overuse.

Rosemary essential oil is refreshing and stimulating to the circulation.

Tea tree essential oil helps skin conditions such as athlete's foot, acne, and warts; it's antifungal, antiseptic, and antiviral.

Thyme essential oil helps relieve chest infections and infected wounds.

LOTIONS, LINIMENTS, SALVES, AND CREAMS

Creams are mixtures of oil and water with a little wax added for body and texture. Many include an emulsifier such as borax, which prevents the oil and water from separating. Some substances add texture as well. Lotions are similar, but lighter and more liquid.

In these preparations, the water and oil phases are broken down to minute, separate particles with the aid of a high-speed blender. An emulsifying ingredient holds the particles in that form, yielding a homogenous preparation that appears to be a single substance. By varying the ingredients, you can create those that are astringent, moisturizing, antifungal, antibacterial, or regenerative.

Poison Ivy or Poison Oak Lotion

This lotion works so quickly and thoroughly that anyone suffering the misery of poison ivy or oak will sing its praises.

½ teaspoon salt (2.5 ml)
½ cup water (118 ml)
cosmetic clay
25 drops peppermint oil

Dissolve the salt in the water and add cosmetic clay until the mixture is creamy. Stir in about 25 drops of peppermint oil and apply to the affected area.

For emergencies, add about 30 drops of peppermint oil to a full bottle of calamine lotion and shake well. Apply as needed.

LINIMENT

A liniment is a liquid preparation with a base of oil, alcohol, or a blend of the two for external application. Liniments are often applied with friction to increase blood circulation to an injury; for sore, stiff muscles, you can use a tincture that includes warming or stimulating essential oils, especially wintergreen, camphor, clove, ginger, cayenne, and cinnamon.

Loosen-up Liniment

2 teaspoons castor oil (10 ml)
1 tablespoon glycerin (15 ml)
1 tablespoon aloe vera gel (15 ml)
1 tablespoon cayenne tincture (15 ml)
30 drops cinnamon essential oil

Combine all ingredients in a bottle and shake well. Apply as necessary.

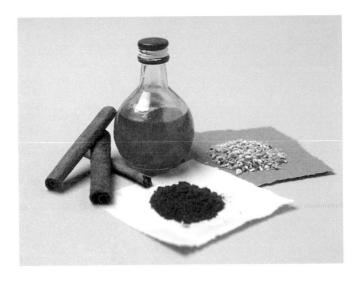

SALVES

Making a salve is a wonderful way to use infused oil. Salve carries the healing properties of the oil, but in solid form; thus it's often more convenient. The salve can be made with a single infused oil or with a combination of several; customizing the salve for individual use is part of the challenge and fun of making it.

Healing Salve

This particularly useful salve incorporates infused oils of yarrow, calendula, and St. John's wort. The salve is designed to reduce inflammation, speed healing, and reduce the possibility of infection when the skin is injured.

½ cup (118 ml) infused oil; use about equal parts of calendula, yarrow, and St. John's wort infused oils
¾ ounce of beeswax (21 grams)
Essential oils for fragrance

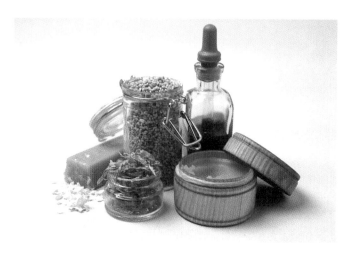

Grate the beeswax. In a saucepan or double boiler, heat the infused oil gently to about 100 degrees Fahrenheit (37°C.). Add grated beeswax slowly, stirring as it melts. Turn off the heat and let the salve cool for a few minutes; add essential oils such as lavender, orange, mint, or thyme as desired.

Test the salve by scooping out a metal spoonful and dipping the back of the spoon in a little bowl of ice water. The salve will harden; if it's too soft, heat the pan again and add a bit more beeswax. If it's too hard, add a bit more oil. Test after each addition to get the product you want.

When you are satisfied with the firmness of the salve, pour it into half-ounce or one-ounce salve jars or other suitable containers. When cool, add lids and label for later use.

Hint: Sometimes when the salve is nearly set, a small crater will appear in the middle of the surface. For a more professional look, add a small amount of hot salve to the hole. When this cools, the hole will be gone.

HEALING CREAMS

Homemade herbal creams can be a luxurious addition to your healing arsenal. Prepared specifically for you, these creams can carry just the right herbs to support healing. Creams, however, can be a little more temperamental than other healing preparations. These tips will help your cream-making more enjoyable and successful.

• Wash all utensils, surfaces, containers, and your hands in antiseptic solution before beginning to make cream, because this combination of ingredients is susceptible to spoilage. Keeping everything as clean as possible will yield a long-lasting cream.

• Creams are composed of an oil phase and a water phase. These two must be prepared and heated separately. When they're mixed, they must be as close as possible to the same temperature, 160 to 175 degrees Fahrenheit (71–79°C.). An emulsifier is required to hold them together in a creamy state. We use ordinary household borax a natural, gentle substance that does the job.

• A handy substitute for the vitamin C powder in the recipes is ascorbic acid, available over the counter at your pharmacy or in the canning area of your grocery store. It serves as a mild preservative. Other possibilities for this purpose include tincture of gum benzoin and grapefruit seed extract added to the water phase, and vitamin E or rosemary oil added to the oil phase.

• Making luscious creams is more an art than a science. Essential oils can provide fragrance and healing qualities, and adding tinctures can customize the cream to your healing needs. Experimentation yields fine combinations that can't be purchased. The combinations suggested for In-A-Hurry Herbal Cream can be used in the other recipes, too.

• Because finished creams are susceptible to spoiling, they're best kept in the refrigerator. Don't dip your finger into the cream; instead, keep it clean by using a little craft stick or a small spoon to scoop it out of the jar.

In-A-Hurry Herbal Cream

To make a quick, useful cream, start with some that the experts have already made: buy a basic cream without fragrance, color, or other additions. You will likely find this in your natural products store, sometimes in bulk.

1 cup of basic cream (237 ml)
Herbal tinctures and essential oils of your choice

Scoop the cream into a the top of a double boiler and heat until it liquifies, usually about 100 degrees F. (37°C.). Stir in up to 20 drops essential oils for their fragrance or healing properties. Add up to one tablespoon of a single tincture or combined tinctures. Stir well, let cool, and return to jar. Suggested combinations:

Antiseptic cream: Thyme or tea tree essential oils to heal cuts and infections.

Damage-control cream: Add rosemary essential oil and vitamin E oil to help the skin heal from sun damage.

Soothing cream: Add witch hazel tincture or calendula tincture to soothe minor burns and itching.

Pain-relieving cream: Add cayenne for a cream to massage into sore muscles, herpes sores, and shingles.

Sprain cream: Add tinctures of arnica and/or St. John's wort to rub on areas that are bruised, strained, or sprained.

For a sweeter-smelling cream, try an equal blend of orange, grapefruit, lemon, and lavender essential oils added to the basic cream.

Skin Protection Cream

This cream prevents drying and chapping.

OIL PHASE:

1 ounce beeswax (28 g)
1 ounce coconut oil (28 g)
4 ounces almond oil (118 ml)
10–20 drops essential oil for scent

WATER PHASE:

2 ounces plain water or scented water
such as rose or orange (59 ml)
2 ounces glycerin (59 ml)
1 teaspoon borax (5 ml)
½ teaspoon vitamin C powder (2.5 ml)

Heat oils and beeswax in a pan; add essential oil when warm. In another pan, heat the water, glycerin, borax, and vitamin C powder. Both phases should be about 160 to 175 degrees Fahrenheit (71–79°C.).

Place the water-phase ingredients in a blender and turn on high. Through the opening in the blender-jar cap, dribble in the hot oil phase. When thoroughly mixed, pour warm cream into jars. Cool and cap.

Light Almond Oil Cream

This light cream soothes the skin.

OIL PHASE:

1 tablespoon beeswax (15 ml)
1 ½ teaspoons coconut oil (8 ml)
1 cup almond oil (237 ml)
10-20 drops essential oil

WATER PHASE:

½ cup water (118 ml)
½ cup aloe vera gel (118 ml)
4 tablespoons glycerin (60 ml)
1 teaspoon borax (5 ml)
1 teaspoon vitamin C (5 ml)

Heat oils and beeswax in one pan; when they're melted, add the essential oil. Heat the water, aloe vera, glycerin, borax, and vitamin C in a separate pan. Both phases should be about 160 to 175 degrees Fahrenheit (71–79°C.).

Put water phase into the blender; at high speed, dribble in the hot oil phase. When thoroughly mixed, pour the cream into jars. Cool and cap.

Ginger-Cayenne Oil Heating Cream

Here's help for muscle aches and pains.

OIL PHASE:

2 teaspoons beeswax (10 ml)
1 tablespoon coconut oil (15 ml)
4 tablespoons cayenne infused oil (60 ml)
10-15 drops wintergreen essential oil

WATER PHASE:

2 tablespoons ginger tincture (30 ml)
2 tablespoons water (30 ml)
2 tablespoons aloe vera (30 ml)
½ teaspoon borax (2.5 ml)
¼ teaspoon vitamin C (1.25 ml)

In a small pan, heat the ginger tincture on medium heat to evaporate as much alcohol as possible without scorching the valuable residue. Then add the water, aloe vera gel, borax, and vitamin C. Heat the beeswax and coconut oil in another pan until melted. Mix the cayenne and wintergreen oils together and add.

When both phases are 160 to 175 degrees Fahrenheit (71–79°C.), pour water phase into a blender set at high speed. Dribble in the oil phase. When thoroughly mixed, pour the cream into jars. Cool and cap.

St. John's Wort Oil-Echinacea Cream

Minor burns, infections, cuts, and rashes are helped by this formula.

OIL PHASE:

2 teaspoons beeswax (10 ml)
1 tablespoon coconut oil (15 ml)
4 tablespoons St. John's wort infused oil (60 ml)
10 drops essential oil of your choice (lavender works well)

WATER PHASE:

2 tablespoons echinacea tincture (30 ml)
2 tablespoons water (30 ml)
2 tablespoons aloe vera gel (30 ml)
¼ teaspoon borax (1.25 ml)
¼ teaspoon vitamin C (1.25 ml)

In a small pan, heat the echinacea tincture on medium heat to evaporate as much alcohol as possible without scorching the valuable residue. Then add the water, aloe vera gel, borax, and vitamin C.

Heat the beeswax and coconut oil in another pan until melted. Mix the St. John's wort infused oil and essential oil together and stir in; heat until warm. Both phases should be about 160 to 175 degrees Fahrenheit.

Put water phase into the blender; at high speed, dribble in the hot oil phase. When thoroughly mixed, pour the cream into jars. Cool and cap.

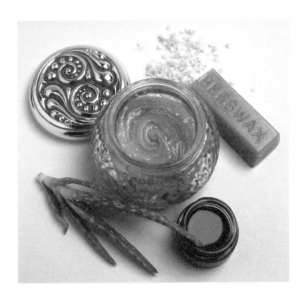

Antifungal Cream

Use this handy cream for athlete's foot, ringworm, or other common fungal infections.

OIL PHASE:

2 teaspoons beeswax (10 ml)
1 tablespoon coconut oil (15 ml)
4 tablespoons almond oil (60 ml)
10-20 drops tea tree essential oil

WATER PHASE:

> *1 tablespoon thyme tincture (15 ml)*
> *1 tablespoon bloodroot tincture (15 ml)*
> *2 tablespoons water (30 ml)*
> *2 tablespoons aloe vera gel (30 ml)*
> *½ teaspoon borax (2.5 ml)*
> *¼ teaspoon vitamin C powder (1.25 ml)*

In a small pan, warm the tinctures on medium heat to evaporate as much alcohol as possible without scorching the valuable residue. Then add the water, aloe vera gel, borax, and vitamin C.

In another pan, mix the almond oil, coconut oil, and the grated beeswax. Heat to melt and add essential oil.

Both phases should be about 160 to 175 degrees Fahrenheit. Pour water phase into blender and turn on high. Slowly dribble the oil phase into the blender. When thoroughly mixed, pour the cream into jars. Cool and cap.

Table 1. Solvent mixes and herb/solvent proportions

| Herb | Part Used | Tinctures | | Infused Oil | Water: Infusion (I) light decoction (LD) decoction (D) |
		Tincture Solvent: % 190-proof alcohol/% water, by volume	Herb: Solvent ratio by volume.		
Arnica	flowers, fresh	100/0	max*	max*	—
Artichoke	leaf, fresh	85/15	max	—	LD
Artichoke	leaf, dried	65/35	1:6	—	LD
Astragalus	dried, prepared root	55/45	1:5	—	D
Black cohosh	dried rhizome	65/35	1:4	—	D
Blue cohosh	dried rhizome	75/25	1:4	—	D
Burdock	dried root	55/45	1:5	max	D
Calendula	dried flowers	100/0	1:5	max	I
Calendula	fresh root	80/20	1:5	—	D
California poppy	dried whole plant	80/20	1:4	—	D
Cayenne	dried fruit	100/0	1:4	max	
Chamomile, German	dried flowers	80/20	1:5	max	D
Chamomile, German	fresh flowers	100/0	max	max	I
Chamomile, Roman	dried flowers	80/20	1:5	max	I
Chamomile, Roman	fresh flowers	100/0	max	max	I
Chicory	dried root	60/40	1:4	—	D
Cinnamon	dried bark	85/0/15	1:4	max	LD

* maximum saturation; that is, as much herb as can be combined in the liquid.

| Herb | Part Used | Tinctures | | Infused Oil | Water: Infusion (I) light decoction (LD) decoction (D) |
		Tincture Solvent: % 190-proof alcohol/% water, by volume	Herb: Solvent ratio by volume.		
Cinnamon	dried twigs	80/20	1:5	max	D
Comfrey	dried leaves	50/50	1:5	max	LD
Cramp Bark	dried bark	80/10/10	1:4	—	LD
Cumin	seed	80/20	1:4	—	—
Dandelion	dried root	60/40	1:4	—	D
Dong quai	dried root	80/20	1:4	max	D
Echinacea angustifolia	dried root	60/40	max	—	LD
Echinacea purpurea	fresh flowers, leaves	50/50	max	—	I
Elder	dried flowers	50/50	1:5	—	I
Elder	fresh flowers	80/20	max	—	I
Elder	dried fruits	40/60	max	—	LD
Eucalyptus	dried leaves	85/15	1:4	—	I
Eyebright	dried herb	70/30	1:5	max	I
Fennel	seed	85/15	1:4	—	I
Fenugreek	seed	40/60	1:4	—	D
Feverfew	dried herb	75/25	1:5	—	I
Feverfew	fresh herb	100/0	max	—	I
Ginger	dried rhizome	85/15	1:5	max	D
Ginger	fresh rhizome	100/0	max	—	D
Ginseng	dried root	50/50	1:5	—	D
Ginseng, American	root, dried	50/50	1:5	—	D
Ginseng, Siberian	dried rhizome	85/15	1:4	—	D
Goldenseal	dried rhizome	75/25	1:3	—	LD
Goldenseal	fresh rhizome	100/0	max	—	I

| Herb | Part Used | Tinctures | | Infused Oil | Water: Infusion (I) light decoction (LD) decoction (D) |
		Tincture Solvent: % 190-proof alcohol/% water, by volume	Herb: Solvent ratio by volume.		
Gotu kola	dried leaves	65/35	max	—	LD
Hawthorn	fresh flowers & twigs	100/0	max	—	I
Hawthorn	dried fruit	65/35	1:5	—	D
Hops	dried strobiles	80/20	1:7	max	I
Hops	fresh strobiles	100/0	max	—	I
Horehound	dried flowering tops	85/15	1:5	—	I
Horsetail	dried herb	50/50	1:5	—	LD
Kava Kava	dried rhizome	95/0	1:3	—	LD
Lavender	dried flowering spikes	80/20	1:5	max	I
Lavender	fresh flowering spikes	100/0	max	max	I
Lemon balm	fresh herb	85/15	1:5	max	I
Licorice	dried root	65/35	1:4	—	D
Ligustrum	dried fruit	60/40	1:4	—	D
Linden	dried flowers	60/40	1:5	—	I
Marshmallow	dried root	50/50	1:5	—	D
Mugwort	dried herb	85/15	1:6	max	LD
Mullein	dried leaf	65/45	1:6	—	LD
Mullein	fresh flowers	85/15	max	max	I
Mustard	seed	55/45	1:4	—	—
Oatstraw	dried spikelets	100/0	max	—	D
Oregon grape root	dried rhizome	75/25	1:4	—	LD
Peppermint	dried herb	85/15	1:5	max	I
Red clover	dried flower heads	60/40	1:5	—	I

| Herb | Part Used | Tinctures | | Infused Oil | Water: Infusion (I) light decoction (LD) decoction (D) |
		Tincture Solvent: % 190-proof alcohol/% water, by volume	Herb: Solvent ratio by volume.		
Reishi	dried mushrooms	85/15	1:8	—	D
Rosemary	dried herb	80/20	1:5	max	I
Sage	dried herb	85/15	1:6	max	I
Self-heal	dried flowering spikes	85/15	1:5	—	D
Spearmint	fresh herb	85/15	1:5	max	I
St. John's wort	fresh flowering tops	100/0	max	max	LD
St. John's wort	dried flowering tops	80/20	1:5	max	I
Stinging nettles	dried root	65/45	max	—	D
Sweet clover	dried herb	80/20	1:5	—	I
Thyme	dried herb	85/15	1:5	max	I
Turmeric	dried rhizome	80/20	1:5	—	D
Usnea	dried herb	100/0	1:5	—	D
Valerian	dried rhizome	80/20	1:4	—	LD
Vitex	dried fruit	85/15	1:4	—	LD
White oak	dried bark	75/25	1:4	—	D
White willow	dried bark	65/45	1:4	—	LD
Wild ginger	dried rhizome	80/20	1:10	max	I
Wild yam	rhizome	65/45	1:4	—	D
Witch hazel	dried bark	80/20	1:4	—	LD
Yarrow	dried herb	85/15	1:5	—	I
Yellow dock	dried root	80/20	1:4	—	D
Yerba santa	leafy shoots	100/0	1:5	—	LD

RESOURCE DIRECTORY

Medicinal Herb Plants, Seeds, and Roots for Gardening

Elixir Farm Botanicals, LLC
Brixey, MO 65618
(417) 261-2393

Specializes in Chinese medicinal herbs and roots such as ginseng, astragalus, and fo-ti. Also supplies medicinal herbs indigenous to North America. Catalog: $2.

Horizon Herbs
P. O. Box 69
Williams, OR 97544
(800) 545-7392

Carries seeds for various medicinal plants, including several echinacea varieties, plantain varieties, gotu kola, and ginseng. Growing guide and catalog, 64 pages, free.

Bulk Herb Suppliers

Aphrodisia
62 Kent Street
Brooklyn, NY 11222
(800) 221 6898

Bulk herbs, including medicinals, spices, and essential oils. Free catalog.

Frontier Herb Co-Op
P. O. Box 299
Norway, IA 53218
(800) 669-3275

Wide selection of bulk herbs, some certified organic; herbal products including soaps and oils. Free catalog.

Mountain Rose Herbs
20818 High Street North
North San Juan, CA 95960
(800) 879-3337

Bulk herbs, many certified organic, organic roses, original medicinal tea formulations.

Mushrooms for Medicinal Use

North American Reishi, Ltd.
P. O. Box 1780
Gibsons, British Columbia
V0N 1V0
Canada
(604) 886-7799

Suppliers of reishi, shiitake, maitake, and cordyceps mushrooms and powdered extracts; also publications about medicinal uses of mushrooms. Minimum purchase required.

Essential Oil Suppliers

Simpler's Botanicals
P. O. Box 2534
Sebastopol, CA 95473
(800) 652-7646
Essential oils, extracts, facial products, infused oils, carrier oils, salves, and body-care products.

Beeswax, Oils, Herbs, Jars

Jean's Greens Herbal Tea Works
119 Sulphur Springs Rd.
Newport, NY 13416
(888) 845-8327

Way of Life
1210 41st Avenue
Capitola, CA 95010
(408) 464-4113
Bulk herbs, full range of vitamin and nutritional supplements, body-care products.

Food Dehydrators

Mountain Home Basics
P. O. Box 1834
Gaylord, MI 49734
(800) 572-9549
Offers two models of Excaliber food dehydrators with thermostat controls as well as grain mills and other products useful to those who like to be self-sufficient.

Grain Alcohol

McCormick Distilling Co.
1 McCormick Lane
Weston, MO 64098
(888) 640-4041
Minimum purchase of four gallons of alcohol required; delivery takes five to seven days.

Herb Press

Kedco
564 Smith St.
Farmingdale, NY 11735
(516) 454-7800 (in NY)
(800) 654-9988
(outside NY state)
This sturdy, manually operated press features a stainless-steel reservoir, spigot and basket. Rubber base reduces sliding. Excellent capacity makes light work of finishing oils and tinctures.

Juicers

Green Power and Champion juicers
Sweetwater Spring
1950 N. 21st St.
Grand Junction, CO 81501
(970) 245-2294

INDEX

Aches 'n Pains Oil 100
acne 17, 91, 92, 101
allergies 15, 33, 91
aloe vera 91, 103, 109, 110, 111
anti-inflammatory 31, 48
antibiotic effects 26, 31, 44, 65, 81, 95
antifungal effects 44, 68, 101, 111
Antifungal Cream 111
antiseptic 30, 32, 34, 68, 101
antiviral effects 20, 26, 28, 35, 44, 77, 81, 89, 101
anxiety 17, 22, 27, 46, 48
arnica 17, 43, 100, 107, 113
arthritis 15, 26, 31, 33, 39, 44, 45, 46, 89, 101
artichoke 86, 113
astragalus 43, 79, 86, 113
astringent 26, 32, 33, 91
Basic Decoction 72
Basic Dried Tea 84
Basic Infusion 70
Bedtime Bath Tea 87
black cohosh 36, 80, 113
blue cohosh 11, 80, 113
boils 21, 29, 44, 92
breast-feeding 15, 25, 27, 32
bruises 17, 32, 107
burdock 17, 21, 38, 80, 113
burns 17, 24, 31, 74, 97, 99, 107, 110
calendula 16, 17, 22, 48, 88, 89, 91, 104, 107, 113
Calendula Infused Oil 74
California poppy 17, 22, 113
Calming After-Dinner Tea 78
cayenne 16, 17, 22, 52, 103, 107, 109, 113

chamomile 17, 20, 32, 30, 48, 70, 71, 76, 78, 87, 89, 101, 113
chicory 38, 113
cinnamon 43, 52, 67, 67, 95, 103, 114
circulation 23, 26, 31, 35, 39, 45, 52, 68, 96, 101, 103
Cleansing Tea 77–78
Cold and Flu Brew 77
cold sores 16, 29
colds 16, 20, 25, 30, 32, 35, 44, 52, 59, 88, 98
colic 52, 70, 71
comfrey 23, 114
congestion 16, 20, 30, 44, 98
cough 16, 27, 30, 32, 44, 68, 97
cramp bark 80, 114
cramps 17, 23, 45, 68, 70
cramps, menstrual 48, 71
cream, variations 105–107
cumin 76, 114
cuts 17, 31, 92, 97, 107, 110
dandelion 11, 17, 24, 38, 51, 66, 114
decoctions 58–60, 72
decongestant 23, 44, 52, 77, 68, 72, 81
digestion 27, 30, 39, 43, 45, 52, 71, 86
dong quai 81, 114
earache 26, 30, 99
Earache Oil 99
echinacea 11, 16, 17 20, 24, 59, 75, 77, 82, 88, 93, 94, 110, 114
Echinacea Tincture 75
Echinacea-Orange Glycerite 93
elder 44, 77, 114
equipment 53–56
essential oil 60, 68, 69, 81, 87, 93, 94, 100,

101, 104, 106, 107, 108, 109, 110, 111
eucalyptus 16, 81, 68, 81, 89, 95, 114
Eye-Love-Herbs Compress Tea 90
eyebright 90, 114
eyewash 27, 33, 90
fennel 25, 76, 78, 81,114
fenugreek 44, 78, 81, 114
fever 16, 20, 40, 44
feverfew 16, 25, 66, 71, 114
flu 20, 25, 30, 35, 59, 77, 98
garlic 16, 20, 26, 40, 52, 66, 99
gas pains 25, 30, 45, 68
ginger 16, 17, 28, 41, 45, 51, 52, 78, 86, 88, 103, 114
Ginger-Cayenne Oil Heating Cream 109
ginseng 36, 45, 53, 62, 79, 86, 114
glycerite 62–63, 92–93
goldenseal 17, 26, 36, 90, 114
gotu kola 88, 91, 115
hawthorn 38, 71, 115
headache 16, 48, 101
Healing Salve 104
Healthy Skin Bath Tea 88
hemorrhoids 40, 46, 73
herbs 41–49
herpes lesions 89, 107
hoarseness 82
hops 27–28, 77, 115
horehound 27, 94, 115
Horehound and Orange Cough Syrup 94
horsetail 84, 85, 115
hypertension (high blood pressure) 27, 46, 52
immune system 15, 20, 25, 43, 45
Immune-Support Tea 79
In-A-Hurry Herbal

Cream 107
infection 17, 25, 26, 33, 43, 45, 89, 92, 96, 97, 90, 101, 104, 107, 110
inflammation 23, 44, 45, 46. 52, 70, 72, 77, 81, 92, 97, 104
infused oil 22, 23, 26, 29, 30, 32, 60–61, 73, 110
infusions 57–60
insect bites 29, 31, 88, 92
insomnia 17, 48, 71
irritable bowel syndrome 23, 24, 29, 30, 46, 48
kava kava 17, 41, 46, 79, 115
lavender 28, 68, 71, 80, 87, 88, 101, 115
laxative 29, 34, 44, 45, 46, 72
lemon balm 16, 20, 28, 59, 66, 71, 76, 78, 82, 87, 89, 115
licorice 16–17, 46, 67, 72, 76, 78, 79, 80, 81, 82, 85, 94, 115
Light Almond Cream 108–109
ligustrum 79, 115
liniment 23, 103
linden 78, 79, 87, 115
liver 24, 34, 39, 44, 77
Loosen-Up Liniment 103
marshmallow 29, 71, 115
Menopause Tea 80
migraine 16, 26, 66, 71
Moon-Cycle Tea 80
mugwort 71, 115
mullein 16, 29, 39, 99, 115
muscle pain 16, 31, 89, 100, 101, 107, 109
mustard 98, 115
Mustard Plaster 98
nausea 28, 30, 39, 45, 52, 71
oatstraw 78, 79, 115

Onion Poultice 97
Oregon grape root 11, 92, 115
pain 22, 40, 46, 68, 96
peppermint 17, 20, 30, 42, 68, 71, 76, 77, 78, 81, 91, 95, 102, 115
plantain 17, 31, 39, 73, 85, 88, 92, 97
Plantain Poultice 97
Poison Ivy or Poison Oak Lotion 102
poultice 21, 35, 39, 96
pregnancy 15, 22, 23, 26, 27, 31, 32, 33, 35, 39, 40, 44, 45, 48, 59, 71
Quick Plantain Infused Oil 73
rash 17, 24, 33, 74, 89, 91, 110
Rash Compress Tea 91
red clover 37, 39, 71, 115
reishi 79, 116
rosemary 31, 66, 68, 89, 101, 107, 116
sage 16, 32, 68, 82, 94, 116
self-heal 40, 116
shingles 29, 107
Skin Protection Cream 108
Sleep Deep Tea 76–77
sore throat 16, 30, 32, 34, 40, 59
sprain 17, 24, 43, 100, 107
St. John's wort 17, 32, 40, 46, 76, 91, 104, 107, 110, 116
St. John's Wort Infused Oil 100
St. John's Wort-Echinacea Cream 110
stevia 67, 77, 78, 79, 81, 95
stinging nettle 33, 40, 80, 84, 85, 116
Strengthen-the-Middle

Dried Tea 86
stress 20, 45, 48
Stress-Buster Tea 79
sunburn 33, 88, 89, 107
Talking Herbs: A Soothing Throat Gargle 82
tea tree oil 68, 101, 107
tea 57–89
Three-Seed Tea 76
thyme 16, 20, 34, 59, 68, 81, 89, 94, 95, 101, 107, 111, 116
tincture 21, 22, 23, 26, 27, 29, 31, 61–62, 75
tonic 26, 30, 31, 32, 33, 39, 45, 71
turmeric 46–47, 52, 116
ulcer 17, 24, 29, 32, 46, 100
urinary tract infection 29, 31, 34, 46, 71
usnea 82, 116
valerian 16, 17, 46, 48, 76, 116
varicose veins 35, 40
Vitamineral Blend Dried Tea 85
vitex berries 80, 116
white oak 91, 116
wild ginger 116
wild yam 80, 116
willow 16, 40, 116
Winter Inhalation 81–82
wintergreen 16, 88, 101, 103
witch hazel 82, 91, 107, 116
Wound and Acne Compress Tea 92
yarrow 17, 20, 34, 41, 77, 89, 92, 104, 116
yeast infection 22, 27, 34
yellow dock 34, 72, 116